ADVANCED PARENTING

ADVANCED PARENTING

ADVICE FOR HELPING KIDS THROUGH DIAGNOSES, DIFFERENCES, AND MENTAL HEALTH CHALLENGES

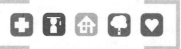

KELLY FRADIN, MD

balance

NEW YORK   BOSTON

Balance
Hachette Book Group
1290 Avenue of the Americas
New York, NY 10104
grandcentralpublishing.com
twitter.com/grandcentralpub

First Edition: April 2023

Balance is an imprint of Grand Central Publishing. The Balance name and logo are trademarks of Hachette Book Group, Inc. The publisher is not responsible for websites (or their content) that are not owned by the publisher.

Library of Congress Cataloging-in-Publication Data

Names: Fradin, Kelly, MD, author.
Title: Advanced parenting : advice for helping kids through diagnoses, differences, and mental health challenges / Kelly Fradin.
Description: First edition. | New York, NY : Balance, 2023. | Includes index. | Summary: "Any parent or teacher who has ever walked out of a concerning appointment with their child's doctor or teacher has experienced a heady mix of emotions—fear, love, confusion, concern, sadness, and perhaps even anger. While every parent hopes for a healthy child, the reality is that children face many common challenges, including medical issues like ADHD, asthma, food allergies, autism, school failure, depression, and developmental delays, throughout their formative years. As the role of a parent becomes one of a caregiver, it can be overwhelming for parents and children alike, particularly if money, time, access, or any combination of those are in short supply. As a balm, Dr. Kelly Fradin offers Advanced Parenting, based on her experience as a complex-care pediatrician. In this crucial guide, parents will find empathy and support as well as evidence-based practical guidance. Of greatest import is the need for tools with which to manage the emotional stress that comes from having a child who deviates from the norm, as well as coping with uncertainty and navigating the business of care. Readers will discover ways to optimize the outcomes for their family and make their day-to-day life easier. Advanced Parenting will help families from the beginning of their journey, beginning with recognizing when a child needs help, accepting the implications of a challenge, obtaining a correct diagnosis, learning about the issue, building a treatment team and coming up with a comprehensive plan. Dr. Fradin explores how a child struggling can affect the entire family dynamic including the parent's relationships and the siblings overall well-being, and with her experience as a complex care pediatrician, she will help parents avoid common mistakes. Parents will feel seen, supported, and better prepared to be both a parent and a caregiver"— Provided by publisher.
Identifiers: LCCN 2022053112 | ISBN 9781538722466 (hardcover) | ISBN 9781538722480 (ebook)
Subjects: LCSH: Parents of problem children. | Parenting. | Problem children—Psychology.
Classification: LCC HQ773 .F73 2023 | DDC 649/.15—dc23/eng/20221107
LC record available at https://lccn.loc.gov/2022053112

ISBNs: 978-1-5387-2246-6 (hardcover), 978-1-5387-2248-0 (ebook)

Printed in the United States of America

LSC-C

Printing 2, 2023

To all the parents who feel overwhelmed by what they face,
and to my husband, Bill, who made this book possible

Contents

Introduction

One sunny day in 2014, I was riding the New York City subway back from the Children's Hospital at Montefiore, where I was working as an attending in the pediatric complex-care group. Our group of pediatricians, nurses, social workers, and care coordinators supported children with severe medical conditions. Only children facing a severe, life-limiting condition such as an organ transplant, congenital heart disease, or chronic respiratory failure requiring long-term use of a breathing tube or ventilator could qualify for the program. We also accepted children who had two less-severe medical conditions—we wouldn't take a child with *just* inflammatory bowel disease or *just* cerebral palsy, but if your child had both, it was likely that they would need our support. For the family's convenience and continuity of care, we also took care of these children's siblings.

This day had been a tough day in a tough week, and a hospitalized patient was not improving. Her underlying genetic disorder and associated medical comorbidities had led to malnourishment. Her poor nutrition had led her to have difficulty with the healing of the skin surrounding her feeding tube, her feeding tube troubles were worsening her malnutrition, and she had just gotten a cold, limiting our ability to do much of anything until her fever subsided and her need for supplemental oxygen decreased. At an hour-long meeting, in which I worked with her family to help coordinate her care, there had been raised voices and tears as they grappled to understand why this was happening, why now, and how to make the best plan with conflicting input from the surgeons, nutritionists, gastroenterologists, and others involved in the case.

A New Field

The field of complex-care pediatrics is relatively small and growing. Its objective is to bring families the support they need through a variety of models. In our model of care at the Children's Hospital, we took on the full primary care role for these chronically ill children *and* their healthy siblings. We had pediatricians who offered longer visits, and we also provided more nursing, social work, and nutrition assistance in advocating for these families. These resources allowed us to provide continuity of care when our patients were in the hospital or emergency room, which happened often; to support finding appropriate school environments; to ensure their homes were well-equipped and accessible; and to provide routine primary care in the clinic. Other models of complex care may work differently; in more rural areas, complex-care pediatricians often help in a consultative role supporting pediatricians in developing an annual care plan. Some states offer care coordination programs with nursing or social work resources through insurance or Medicaid plans.

Working in complex care many days has the same feel as being a regular pediatrician—I work to support children and families. Sometimes the stakes are higher and more intense and the conditions more complex, but despite carrying more diagnoses or having more healthcare needs, at the end of the day it's still about helping children and their families. One bright side of the increased frequency of visits is that as the pediatrician, I have the opportunity to get to know the family better. On average, the children in my practice came to my office around four to eight times a year and I saw them through one to two hospital stays in addition. Because of the time we spent together and the privilege of getting to really know the patients in my care, these families taught me much of what I know as a pediatrician about what it's like to face a challenge.

On particularly difficult days I appreciated having time to decompress and process the day on the way home from work. This day I sat on the subway, scrolling through social media and rethinking my work with this family and how I could do more to help them, when a friend from my neighborhood called. At just age two, her son had been diagnosed with asthma after several colds involving extreme wheezing. She was struggling to understand why this was happening, why now, and how to make the best plan with input from her husband, mother-in-law, pediatrician, and new pulmonologist. My first thought was that mild asthma is *easy* compared to what I do day to day with *really* sick kids. Still, as I talked through things with her, I could not ignore the similarities in these families' struggles.

These children were in wildly different places—one was hospitalized and threatened with admission to the ICU, and the other was at the playground; each experienced entirely unrelated problems, one with a genetic diagnosis and one more likely triggered by environmental factors—and yet the parents were coping with similar stress. How could they process their situation, make sense of it, and move forward? I knew I could help them both. I could help them understand and research what they faced, find resources that they needed to make decisions with confidence, and put together a team approach to be proactive and preventive in the future with their child's health.

But at the same time, I thought, this work does not fit within a fifteen-minute visit or a message sent through a health-care portal. I wondered why the systems weren't set up to better support these families. Parenting is hard. Because we care so deeply for our children, as parents we want things to be perfect. As a parent, you want things to go as planned. You want to be prepared for every developmental change and anticipate your child's needs to properly support them. But parenting is *even harder* when things do not follow a typical trajectory.

When your child deviates from the typical developmental pathway or when they are struggling with their physical or mental health, everyday challenges become much more intense. The fear and the uncertainty can be overwhelming. For parents raising children with these additional needs, there seem to be, oddly, fewer resources. While parents are drowning in parenting content and consuming it at an all-time high, most parenting advice is geared toward average children facing typical challenges, from getting a baby to sleep to helping a teen with their nascent independence.

Why is it that we leave so many parents adrift for what is, for many, the hardest part of their lives? Historically, families with children with health challenges have faced stigma. Though we are thankful to live in a more inclusive society, and though we know that nearly one-third of children experience chronic medical conditions, the available resources haven't caught up. There is a growing awareness that some parents need access to additional caregiving skills—advanced parenting skills that can help them support their children through a challenge.

The Challenge vs. The Problem

I use the term "challenge" in an intentionally inclusive way. If your child has a broken leg, you will have a hopefully short-term challenge, but in that time, you will still need to establish a pain-control plan; reorganize your household; communicate with school, childcare, and sports; and navigate the medical complex to receive treatment that promotes healing. You'll have to support your child's coping and recovery after the cast comes off. Although health-care providers see injuries like this every day and may consider them small potatoes, when it happens to your child, it can feel overwhelming considering that you now have to devote time and energy you likely don't have and didn't expect to spend on an emergency. But that time and energy has to come from somewhere.

Perhaps, though, you are helping your child who has a physical disability like cerebral palsy—their muscle coordination is impaired due to abnormal brain development early in life. This is a long-term challenge, which also requires you to develop a pain-control plan; reorganize your household; communicate with school, childcare, and sports; and navigate the medical complex to get treatment to promote healing. You'll have to support your child's coping and recovery. Is it the same as a child who has "just" broken their leg? No, absolutely not. But the skills you need to navigate these very different issues are similar.

When I began considering writing this book nearly ten years ago, I thought about helping a family with a problem. Some challenges families face feel like problems—chronic allergies and asthma, a heart defect that needs a repair, a behavioral disturbance that needs to be controlled to prevent injury, or a hemangioma (strawberry birthmark) that needs intervention. If you were drawn to this book, you likely identify what you're facing as a problem—a negative disturbance that needs a remedy. That's a completely valid and important reason to have sought this book out, and you will find help within its pages.

There's another group of parents and caregivers who will find this book useful. Your child may struggle with anxiety, hyperactivity, autism, learning disabilities, or a genetic diagnosis. I need to make plain that viewing these conditions as "problems" needing "fixing" propagates stigma. Our society, including people like me, has a deeply ingrained ableism that assumes people with disabilities are somehow "less than." Just as racism or sexism leads to harmful stereotypes and systems of exclusion, so does ableism. Some differences are part of who we are, and some of our differences should be welcomed and embraced rather than fixed. We may still need a plan or support to navigate our own path forward when it deviates from the default standard plan, but we are seeking to live and thrive *with* the diagnosis rather than fix it.

While no word is perfect, my hope is that "challenge" has a more positive connotation. The goal is to not just fix or remedy a problem, but to more comprehensively support the entire family, the children and the parents, to find peace and joy in their lives despite any challenges they face. A challenge represents an opportunity for growth; our difficulties can differentiate us and make us who we are; our diagnoses are part of us in a way that can enrich and enhance the way we experience life. Perhaps I see this so vividly because I've faced a few health-related challenges myself.

An Early Diagnosis

One night, right before Mother's Day when I was four years old, I fell out of bed. The minor fall led to massive pain, and urgent surgery for suspected appendicitis. The surgeons didn't find an infected appendix, but they did find internal bleeding that could not be explained by an innocent fall. They accused my parents of child abuse and pressured my parents for consent to remove my bleeding kidney. My parents were uneasy with this plan. The rural hospital had no imaging capacity at that time, and none of this made sense. So, they snuck me out a stairwell and took me to Duke Children's Hospital in Durham, North Carolina, where they knew they'd have access to proper resources to support my care. Now, as a pediatrician and a parent myself, I can more clearly understand what my parents went through. Not only did they cope with a child who went from being healthy to sick very quickly, but amidst uncertainty and coercion from medical professionals, they also had the confidence to advocate for another plan.

At Duke, specialists were able to diagnose me with a rare kidney cancer known as Wilms' tumor and made a plan for me to receive world-class treatment. But my family's life turned upside down, as this was hours from our small town, which lacked the medical care I needed. So, my family split up, leaving my dad to stay behind and work to keep our family afloat, while my mom quit her job and moved with me into the Ronald McDonald House at Duke to support me through hospital admissions, chemotherapy, radiation, and surgeries.

Because of my parents' massive efforts, the doctors at Duke Children's Hospital, and the Ronald McDonald House, we made it through. By age six, I was lucky to go into complete remission and was ultimately cured of cancer, and I now lead a more or less healthy life as an adult. But what stuck with me through the experience was the understanding that my cancer journey was so much harder on my mother than it was on me. Yes, I faced needles and surgeries. I started kindergarten bald and with an implanted port to allow for IV chemotherapy. But my mom thought many times she might lose her child. She faced an intense chronic stress that never fully went away. Though I was healthy and in my late thirties, and she was in her early sixties, when the COVID-19 pandemic began, she would call me worried about my well-being. She still saw me as needing extra caregiving attention, even decades after my recovery.

One Size Fits Most

It's precisely because I've seen families facing challenges from so many perspectives—as a pediatrician to thousands of children over the years, as a friend and family member supporting a loved one facing challenges, and as a child and adult with my own challenges—that I have written this book to tackle all aspects of helping your child face a challenge. In part I, we'll discuss understanding what you bring to the challenge and what your priorities are. In part II, we'll discuss how to research and understand the system you're working in and craft a plan with your bigger picture and team in mind. In part III, we'll cover strategies to promote your family's wellness and find joy on your journey. In part IV, we'll focus on ensuring your plan is comprehensive and considering the how to maintain your motivation over the long-term.

While I can't know what challenge led you to pick up this book, the goal is for this guidance to help you to gain confidence and make the right decisions for your family, rather than learn the hard way. Whether your challenge is "small" or "big" or whether you'll only need to make a few changes to your routine or need a real overhaul of your plan informed by new perspectives, hopefully the anecdotes and information in this book will assist you. Maybe your challenge is brand-new and I will introduce you to the world of parents who have faced similar stresses before you, and through them you'll learn the language required to navigate systems to advance your child's care. Maybe your challenge has been going on for years and you have already dealt with many of the topics discussed. Even in that case, I hope this book will prompt you to process what you've been through and consider how it has impacted you and your family. It could be you'll find some ways to improve aspects of your plan, something you could tweak to promote your child's well-being or your well-being as a caregiver. Depending on what you are facing and where you are along your journey, you may find different ways to make the most of this book. It may be most helpful to read straight through the book, which roughly parallels the path of encountering a challenge from beginning to end. Or you may jump around, guided by the table of contents, to find the topics most salient to your family today.

Maybe you haven't encountered a real challenge for your child yet, but you're curious about what you should know when one comes up, or about ways you can be a more empathetic presence in your community supporting families facing challenges. This book tries as much as possible to be inclusive and cover the broad variety of challenges families face, but it's difficult to anticipate the specific diversity of unique situations and experiences. My intentions here are pure—to help in any way I can.

The reason I've designed this book to try to have something for everyone is twofold. First, I recognize that a lot of children face something relatively rare—a genetic diagnosis, a congenital abnormality, a developmental disability, or maybe a kidney cancer like mine, which is diagnosed in around fifty children annually in the US. Many of the main supports accessible to parents are diagnosis driven, so children facing more common diagnoses like asthma, diabetes, or inflammatory bowel disease may find a bigger, more robust support community, unintentionally leaving out those more unique families. Second, parents facing challenges have more in common than they realize. When we focus on these human commonalities, we see what connects us and unites us. Breaking free of the silos of diagnoses—being a "heart kid" facing a congenital heart defect, a parent of a premature infant or parent of a "tubie" (a child fed by feeding tube)—allows us to see that we are all advocating for our children in our local hospitals, schools, and communities and can broaden our support networks. Building these bridges helps us learn from each other and over time can make our communities more supportive and understanding places for everyone.

Regardless of where you are, it's important you understand that you are not alone. Facing a challenge is inherently isolating, especially when your family is dealing with a rare condition or lives in a smaller town. It could be the local doctors and the nearby school have no experience with a child like yours, and you may not know anyone who has ever had to do the things you now do. But as I share these stories, perhaps you'll see that many if not most parents face a challenge that requires these additional advanced parenting skills. It may be that you are facing growth hormone deficiency, and another child has developmental delay and plagiocephaly (a flat head) requiring a helmet, but you both have to do research to process the ever-changing body of knowledge on the condition. You both have to help support your child in coping and gaining skills and independence in their own care. You have to figure out how to work with the school, sports, and babysitters, and continue to support your other children if you have them. While on the surface these children may seem to be fighting very different battles, at a deeper level we are all facing similar dynamics.

Your challenge may seem common, perhaps something like asthma, but the way you are experiencing the challenge may not feel common. Maybe your child is struggling to cope with the trauma of a scary episode, or you struggle to fit in the unpredictability of the condition with the rest of your life. Your experience of this common condition is unique to your family, and often, the standard advice or the fifteen-minute visits with your doctor don't get to the place where you need the most help, leaving you feeling inadequately supported in making the best plan for your child. This book is intended to fill the gaps.

It's in Your Hands

In our current framework, when a parent invests time and energy to support their child through an experience like being born preterm with a long NICU stay, with subsequent multidisciplinary care needs like physical therapy and nutrition, we view it through the lens of victimhood.

Something bad has happened, and a parent is expected to cope with a problem as best they can on their own. This parent just deals and steamrolls through a difficult time, helpless to change the landscape and reduce the hurdles facing their family.

But when we change the dialogue to talk about the agency parents have in the process, we can empower them. For the parent, we can talk about this work as an achievement and see that, despite the challenges, you gain skills that have value in supporting yourself and your child in real and important ways. Instead of passively letting things happen to us and our family, we can attempt to take some control for how we cope and the choices we make along the way—using our voices to advocate for change. We can decide to focus on more than not only getting through difficult times, but also on thriving *despite* difficult times.

When parents learn these advanced parenting skills and start to advocate for what their families need to thrive, it can make a big impact on public health. Parents can drive change in their communities, their schools, their clinics, and their hospital systems to get the resources they need to support their families. With this positive, constructive vision, let's dive in.

PART I

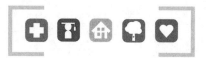

BUILD A SOLID BASE

CHAPTER 1

Understanding Your Reaction to a Problem

My daughter was a quiet baby. Although she was very interactive and social, she wasn't one to babble or coo much. She was born a little premature, and, as a pediatrician, I thought, *I'll just be patient.* But, as a parent, I felt she wasn't developing as I expected, especially compared to her brother. She was not as responsive to speech and environmental noise, and my intuition told me something was wrong. I requested a hearing test at our nine-month visit and the doctor talked me out of it. "She's fine. No ear infections. Normal ear exam. Let's give her a bit more time." My excellent pediatrician felt that her development was within an acceptable range and an additional hearing test wasn't necessary. He wasn't a gatekeeper, and I could have pushed him for a referral, but his opinion was that waiting to see if she started babbling was the less invasive and more appropriate route.

But still, his advice didn't sit right with me. So, a few weeks before her first-year visit, I made my own appointment for a hearing test. In the audiology test room, stuffed monkeys clanged loud cymbals, but my daughter did not respond. It was clear that not only did she have a hearing problem, but it wasn't mild. She had moderately severe hearing loss due to chronic fluid in the middle ear. If I had done as my pediatrician recommended and waited, my daughter would not have had a routine hearing test until entering kindergarten, years later, or until she had failed to reach developmental milestones.

As a pediatrician myself, I completely understand why my pediatrician recommended to wait and see. He made a judgment call about what might have been an unnecessary referral, and he may have also thought that if she did have a hearing problem, the benefit of addressing it then as opposed to three months later was limited. Pediatricians make hundreds of calls like this every day and do their best. But for me, as a parent, this decision about the way in which my daughter interacted with the world seemed much more important. I would rather have wasted my time with an unnecessary referral than to have delayed my daughter's ability to hear and to communicate with her family. After a minor surgery to help the fluid clear, within a week she was babbling, and within a month she had fifty words.

The takeaway here, of course, is that I had all the information. As a pediatrician I knew about hearing tests and speech development. As her mom, I knew her and could compare her development with that of her brother. But still, I almost didn't get her the care she needed because my pediatrician and I both questioned my intuition. At nine months, it's hard to really describe what you see in terms of speech development—how often a baby babbles, how loudly and with what variety of sounds, and how they respond to the sounds in their environment. I presented my doctor with a vague comment—something seemed off and she was quiet. I was concerned. Why did we both dismiss this so quickly?

A parent's intuition can be a very powerful force. As Gavin de Becker describes in *The Gift of Fear*, "We think conscious thought is somehow better, when in fact, intuition is soaring flight compared to the plodding of logic." A parent knows more data about their child than a doctor will ever know—the sound of a tired laugh, the change in color that indicates a coming cold, and how a child will respond in a novel or unfamiliar circumstance. Often, when a parent is worried, there is usually a good reason, even if it's not immediately apparent what it is.

The few months' delay in my daughter's hearing test didn't really matter much, but the story serves to remind you of a simple fact: Your intuition is one of the most important resources you bring to supporting your child facing a challenge. Information, resources, and credentials have value, but nothing supplants just how well you know your child.

That all said, parenting in the twenty-first century can be anxiety inducing. Your gut reaction and your intuition can be very helpful, but parents should be mindful. Your first instinct, taken out of context, can also lead you astray. Our temperaments and prior experiences will influence not only whether we listen to our gut, but also whether, after listening, we take the right steps forward. Our supports—family, educators, physicians, and others in our community—can help us harness the power of our intuition while grounding our instincts in facts and reality.

When you are confronting a challenge, you want to have the *right* plan. But oftentimes, there are many possible paths forward, and there may be more than one that's right for your situation. Before you decide the best way forward, it can be helpful to think about what you bring to the challenge as a parent that will guide your reaction.

What Do You Bring to the Challenge?

Consider as a scenario: You're packing for vacation. Some people pack light—they're flexible; they figure they can pick up what they need at the destination—maybe they forgot something, or perhaps it rains unexpectedly, and they need to purchase an umbrella. Others are inclined to bring everything they could ever possibly need so they can be prepared for any situation. There is nothing intrinsically wrong with either approach. Everyone can have fun and have what they need. But what you show up with will alter your plan. If you show up without what you need, you'll have to go get it. If you show up with a lot of heavy bags, you may not be able to carry them yourself.

Part of the difference in approach depends on differences in who you are. Are you a planner or are you someone who likes to be more spontaneous? Your packing strategy may also reflect your specific situation.

Are you a single twenty-something or a family of five? Maybe your loved one surprised you with this vacation and you didn't get the notice needed to pack. Your decisions about packing may also reflect your state of mind before the trip—if it was the busiest time of your life, you may not have had time to pack. But if you have been thinking about this trip for two years, you may have had a color-coded packing list.

Similarly, when our families approach a challenge, what we bring will vary. You will not be immune to setbacks just because of your carefree disposition, for example, and you will not be "doomed" if you don't have the "right" starting place. Still, the reality of what you bring to the situation will affect your plan.

If you are a family who packs light:

- You may prefer to keep things spontaneous and learn as you go.
- You may have the ability to be nimble as you adapt to the challenge you face.
- You may have been surprised by this challenge.
- You may not know a lot about the particular challenge you face.
- You may not have had prior experiences with children with medical or educational challenges.
- You may be facing a challenge that is less serious or that seems likely to improve quickly.

If you are a family who carries a lot of baggage:

- You may prefer to approach things with abundant planning and research.
- You may have more going on, more kids, more aging loved ones, more work, or more financial stress that requires your attention and makes you less flexible and adaptable.
- You may have had a prior experience with this type of challenge or issues that are similarly serious.

- You may be facing a challenge that is more serious or that is expected to require several interventions or a longer period of attention.

I would argue both families can succeed in facing their challenges, whether they have packed light or packed heavily. If you can have some perspective into what you're showing up with—including the things you perceive as both strengths and weaknesses—you can use that insight to help make the best plan for your family.

It's worth noting that if you experienced the same challenge as your child, you may feel better equipped as a parent. For example, you and your child may have the same learning disability or food allergy. As a parent, you are bringing a lot of valuable firsthand experience and knowledge that can help your family. But you also may be bringing some outdated ideas (things have changed!) and some preconceived notions that may not apply to your child. Maybe your teacher wasn't helpful with your learning disability or you never had a severe allergic reaction. But just because you had those experiences doesn't mean your child will. Sometimes these experiences give you valuable background, vocabulary, and context, but for other families bringing along these experiences is like carrying flip-flops on your ski vacation; they may have been useful for childhood beach trips, but they will be of little use to you on the slopes.

More importantly, you may have unprocessed emotional trauma to unpack. Maybe you were shamed or bullied for the learning issues you faced, or maybe you ended up in the ICU after a severe reaction and almost died. You may find your child's issues trigger painful memories. So, as you try to "enjoy your trip," you'll want to use the learnings that are most useful and find ways to process and heal from the rest. You can draw from what you've experienced to support your child, but you should not allow your past to bar you from understanding what's changed and what's different about your child's situation.

If you are packing light for vacation, you may need to shop when you get there and seek out more resources. If you had never before heard the words "cerebral palsy" or known a child with a developmental disability, and now your child may be diagnosed with one, you may feel like the airline lost your luggage completely. You may not have many preconceived notions or much background in the sort of challenges you face, and that may feel overwhelming. But you can parent effectively even if you may need to do some research and seek out more support to meet the demands of your situation.

As a pediatrician, I often don't know the full family baggage. When I first meet a child with chronic severe headaches, for example, I may not know that their mom has had headaches for years and suffered greatly. It may be difficult for the mother to imagine her child reliving such a negative experience. Or maybe the dad's nephew just bounced between specialists for four months trying dozens of treatments before being diagnosed with a brain tumor, so the family is terrified that their child's headache means a similar fate. Or maybe the parent never really had headache issues and doesn't even keep over-the-counter pain medications in the house. As your family's doctor, I won't really know what kind of support you need as a parent without knowing this context. What I need to know is, where are you coming from?

But I've seen families hold back on this information. Some families think that the pediatrician is only there to support the child—a huge misconception. Pediatricians are advocates for children, positioned to support their growth, development, and health; but in order to accomplish this work, pediatricians are expected to evaluate and support the well-being of the family. The Bright Futures preventive health guidelines by the American Academy of Pediatrics recommend pediatricians make room at every visit to ask open-ended questions about family stressors and gain expertise in utilizing family strengths and community supports to optimize family functioning. It's easiest to see this necessity in the extremes—when a mother has postpartum depression, her mental health is a direct concern for her child. If there is domestic violence or substance abuse in the home, we know the child's health and well-being will be affected. But even in more everyday examples, a pediatrician is responsible for supporting both the parent and the child because caring for the family directly impacts the child's well-being.

Still, some families shy away from opening up about where they are coming from; maybe they are focused on using our limited time on the issue at hand or they do not see how it's relevant. Maybe parents seek to avoid judgment from the medical provider. But speaking with your doctor about the context of your family can be a game changer, particularly when things feel overwhelming or aren't going well.

As fully formed adults, we also bring our attitudes and personalities to parenting, which can be strengths. Maybe you're an extrovert and have a big network of friends to help you. Or maybe you have a voracious appetite for reading books to help you prepare. Maybe you are very intuitive and observe your child intensely. The characteristics that make you the parent that you are can also help you support your family in your own unique way.

Your personality traits can also be weaknesses. Maybe you struggle with organization or you do not have a lot of experience with breaking down big, complex projects. Maybe you're a procrastinator or prone to sweeping hard things under the rug. Maybe you're more of an introvert and don't have a big community of friends to support you.

We all have our blind spots and biases, even in the medical field. Pediatricians have seen rare and terrible illnesses—not because these things are common, but because we see thousands of patients over our careers. For example, I've seen a thousand kids with a stomachache, and only once was it related to a new diagnosis of cancer. For some, this experience leads them to worry excessively about their children's health. Others, like me, cope with this fear by denying or minimizing the possibility that my children could be seriously ill. But, by being aware of our tendency, a paranoid parent can seek extra reassurance, and since I have a bias to dismiss potential problems, I can make a plan to ensure my kids get good care. At the end of my visit with the doctor, I can ask, "Should I be worried about this?" And I can welcome my husband's perspective to round out my own.

In the end, the most important thing you bring to a challenge is the love you have for your child. You care about them more than anyone else in the world. You know them better than anyone else. And so, you're in the best position to help them. Taking an honest look at your strengths and weaknesses, perspectives and biases will prepare you to handle this challenge the best way you can. Self-awareness will help you find the balance you need to become the best advocate for your child. And whatever your background, all parents can find ways to help their children.

Before you go on, take a moment to think about the following:

- What's the biggest strength you bring to helping your child face their challenge?
- What's an area where you feel you could grow or get help?
- How will the background of your day-to-day life affect the unique way you approach things?

Worrying the "Just Right" Amount

So much of the stress I hear about from parents relates to the uncertainty of whether they are on the right track. How do you know if you are too worried, or not worried enough? Say a child's weight hovers right around the edge of where you begin to be concerned about malnutrition. Or a child's development is just a touch slower than what you might expect. Or a baby is just a little fussier than other babies, or a teenager seems more emotional than you'd expect.

We do not want to pathologize our children. We shouldn't think of every little thing as a problem or an emergency. This kind of over-worrying can do more harm than good. At the same time, we do not want to miss an opportunity to find our child the support they need to live their best life. I think of trying to achieve the "just right" amount of concern as like shooting a basketball into a hoop. You want to estimate the proper amount of force you'll need to get the ball the correct distance, and you want to aim for the net.

If you underestimate the challenge and bring too little force, you may not have enough oomph to get to the net. You may not devote energy to discussing the challenge with babysitters, teachers, and doctors who could help. During the delay, your child's condition may worsen.

But on the other hand, if you overestimate the challenge and bring too much force, you may tire yourself out or bang the ball against the backboard and still miss the net. When you devote excessive resources to a challenge, you steal resources from other important areas of your life, which can cause unnecessary anxiety. You may miss some of the joys of parenting. Or children may hear the message that there is something wrong when there isn't.

If you think back to how you've responded to other issues that you've handled in your life, consider if you might have a default response to difficult situations. In high school, for example, when you knew you were heading toward a bad grade, did you avoid the issue and forget about it? Or did you worry a lot, changing your behavior and studying? Have you ever had a situation where you looked back and thought, "Maybe I overreacted?" Our default response to challenges can be part of our temperament. We often trend toward familiar behaviors when it comes to worrying too much or too little.

Now, considering what we've discussed so far, you may want to think about where you fall on the scale between someone who is avoidant and someone who catastrophizes. Some things to consider:

A Parent in Denial

- Others around you seem more concerned about your child's challenge than you are.
- You may find yourself minimizing your child's challenge often.
- You may be seeing the trees instead of the forest.

A Parent Who Panics

- It seems every minor thing is terribly wrong.
- Small problems seem overwhelming.
- Worries seem to crowd your thoughts and your mind is often racing through the worst scenarios.

As you consider your reaction to your child's challenge, take time to investigate whether your reaction is in correct proportion to the scale of the challenge.

It's also important to pause to consider what message you'd like to send to your child and what attitude you'd like your children to have toward their challenge. Your reaction or overreaction will affect how your child understands their challenge. Your response will also affect how your child believes in your ability and their own ability to face this challenge. Between your reaction and your response, there is a space for your best intention. But before you can make use of that space, you have to be honest about what your reaction is and where it's coming from.

Ultimately, please understand that it is possible, even common, that sometimes you will tend toward denying problems and sometimes you will jump toward catastrophic thinking. Both extremes are rooted in love, but at the extremes, either can harm your child. Minimizing the situation can lead to missing opportunities for positive intervention. And panicking can frighten your child and create excessive stress.

Happily, there are specific ways to address each of these tendencies. Finding balance can help you chart a constructive path forward for your family.

Denial

Let me walk you through a relatively common scenario for many pediatricians: Let's say I'm about to see a six-year-old for a sick visit for breathing concerns. He has missed twenty-four days of school in the last year. He has been seen in urgent care twice and has been hospitalized with a severe case of influenza. When I see that he has a diagnosis of asthma and several medications on file, this all makes sense. Asthma is one of the most common chronic medical conditions kids face, and it can be quite difficult to control.

As I enter the room, I would be wondering what factors we may have missed that may have led to our struggles to get his asthma under control. Perhaps he has severe allergies, or perhaps the controller medication wasn't the right choice. The first thing I ask is how his asthma has been recently. His father then furrows his brow and says his son doesn't have asthma.

Now I am confused. Did I look at the wrong chart? I reviewed the facts as I saw them in the chart: prescriptions, ER visits, a hospital stay . . . this is the correct medical history. Had it been one or two encounters for asthma, I would think maybe communication difficulties and poor explanations led Dad to misunderstand. But over a dozen encounters mentioned asthma, and asthma inhalers had been prescribed. The child had a past diagnosis of asthma in each visit, but the dad did not agree. If the breathing problems weren't due to asthma, what were they about? "I don't know," Dad says, "he just gets a bad cough sometimes."

Because this is not my first rodeo, I recognize the parental issue pretty quickly—denial. I have seen the reactions families can have when they face a challenge, and they can have considerable range. When you watch your child day to day, you gain so much information—more than anyone else could possibly have. You see how much they sleep, how they eat, their activity level, and their mood. You see what frustrates them and what brings them joy. You see how they interact with friends in familiar and unfamiliar settings. You have all the data.

This valuable knowledge sets you up to have all the information you need to make a diagnosis, but it doesn't always happen. As parents, we also have a deep need for our children to be all right. We love our children immensely and hate to imagine that things are wrong or that they need additional help. Sometimes we are too close to the situation to see a growing problem or a trend. Sometimes it's much easier to bury our heads in the sand and deny that there is a problem. Denial feels safe and thus is an easy trap to fall into. Over time, I've learned that this denial often stems from fear.

Even as a professional, I'm guilty of this. My child wakes up in a grumpy mood, refuses breakfast, and has a bit of a runny nose. I think about our busy day and I hurry my child along the usual routine. More than once, my husband has had to stop and say, "Hello; our child isn't just grumpy, he's sick." I am too close to the situation and often heavily biased toward wanting everyone to be well for logistic reasons (I don't want to cancel work or school) and for emotional reasons (I just don't want to face the possibility that my babies aren't well).

When I dug further into the aforementioned asthma case, a review of all the common symptoms made it clear he had all the classic signs of asthma. He checked all the boxes, including chronic nighttime cough and shortness of breath when exercising. But the father vehemently denied the diagnosis of asthma. You can imagine how this denial would be a major obstacle in getting the child the help he needed. Before I could help the parent to properly treat the child, I needed him to accept and understand the problem. By not acknowledging the scale of the challenge they faced, the father was having difficulty getting the son the support he needed.

Rather than confronting the dad, I chose to approach the situation with curiosity: "It sounds like you know a lot about asthma. When I hear your son's symptoms, the diagnosis of asthma seems clear to me, but can you tell me what I am missing?" And that's when more of the story came out. The father had childhood asthma that worsened in his teenage years. He had been in intensive care and even on a ventilator for his asthma. "I know asthma is *bad*," he said, "and what he has is not that bad."

This opened up the conversation. As we talked through his experience in contrast to his son's, I could see him visibly relax. Now we could start from common ground. And once I understood where he was coming from, I could provide targeted education about how variable symptoms and severity can be in asthma. I then was able to guide him to see how accepting the diagnosis would help keep his son well.

When he was denying that his son had a problem, the father had been underestimating the need for resources to improve his son's health. Once he accepted the diagnosis of asthma, he could provide the care his child needed to thrive. He could learn that treating asthma did not always mean ventilators, and that asthma does not always mean worsening symptoms over time. He could see that the goal of treatment was not just about avoiding hospital stays. He could see that by treating his son's cough, we could improve his sleep quality and potentially his behavior and school performance. By controlling the asthma, we could improve his son's endurance and even increase his interest in sports and other physical activity.

When I understood the gap between what I saw and what the father saw, I could help so much more. The medication would help to avoid emergency hospital stays and control his son's breathing problems, and also improve the family's quality of life.

Denial can come in many shapes and sizes, but it is the tendency to minimize, ignore, or circumnavigate a challenge that needs to be addressed. Very loving and engaged parents can exhibit tendencies toward denial for valid reasons. We want our child to be well, so sometimes we sweep small signs of trouble under the rug and are the last to identify something as a problem. We see our child change in very gradual ways over a long period of time and sometimes lose the perspective that our child's experience is unusual or abnormal. We are so used to our child and the way our child has always been that we don't always compare our children to what is normative at their age (sometimes for good reason!). The associated reluctance to ask for help and obtain care can do harm. No parent intentionally obstructs their child's care, and often the denial is unconscious.

If you tend toward denial, self-awareness can help you manage your tendencies and provide direct benefits to your child. You could remind yourself to take a closer look or a regular step back to consider issues you tend to avoid. Or you can invite others in your life to remind you and support you when needed. Babysitters, teachers, friends, or family should feel welcome to speak up if they think your child needs more attention or resources.

In our family, I am prone to denial, and my husband is the one who frequently has to nudge me toward taking action. His input is welcome and helpful, even if sometimes I still don't act on it right away. But awareness and improvement—even partial improvement—can still make a positive impact in our child's care.

It's Not Always the End of the World

While denying a problem can delay care and negatively impact the child, it's also true that overreacting to a problem can do harm. Imagine a parent who sees blood in their child's diaper. Without knowledge to interpret this symptom, a parent primed to catastrophize may worry about cancer or a surgical emergency like appendicitis. If the parent is interpreting the situation as a catastrophe, the parent may suffer stress and lose sleep, choosing to seek out a gastroenterologist. They may then have to wait for an appointment, spending money and time to lean on a specialist's expertise to rule out cancer. These steps may not have been necessary and may result in a longer lag time before their child gets appropriate counsel. Similarly, if a parent is concerned about blood in the stool being a sign of a surgical emergency like appendicitis, the parent may run their child to the emergency room. While evaluation at the emergency room might yield a diagnosis, so would a call or visit to the pediatrician with less cost and exposure to viruses and bacteria. Responding this way once in a while might be an expected part of parenting—surely sometimes we overreact—but when overreacting becomes a pattern, it can lead to unnecessary stress, diminished sleep, impaired decision-making, and other consequences.

A parent without the tendency to catastrophize or with a more trusting relationship with their pediatrician may be able to find better care faster and with less cost (and less stress). The pediatrician can help a family determine what blood in the diaper might represent in the context of this child's family and medical history. Most likely, the pediatrician could provide immediate reassurance about cancer and surgical emergencies being unlikely and underlying constipation or milk protein allergy being the most likely possible diagnoses. By partnering with their pediatrician, parents will have individualized support in addressing their concerns and connecting with any needed specialists for interventions.

Imagine another scenario, a child who has limitations in expressive language. This child may be on a different timeline than other children in accomplishing their milestones. A parent who is prone to catastrophizing—imagining only the worst possibilities—may be prone to "give up" on their child and think they may never gain these skills. This attitude may translate into less patience with practicing recommended skills or less motivation to schedule therapy sessions. It's important to understand that this often comes from a good place; a parent may be accepting the child for who they are today. But sometimes fear or trauma leads us to imagine our children's future as more limited than it may be.

The attitudes parents carry about a diagnosis are passed on to their children. When you view your child as having more challenges than they actually do—thinking they are more fragile, more sick, more troubled, more disadvantaged—your child can begin to internalize these messages. Some studies have shown that the extent of these impacts can be wide ranging. Intuitively we understand that catastrophizing is a maladaptive coping pattern, and research has confirmed that adults or children who catastrophize tend to have worse outcomes.

With chronic pain, catastrophizing attitudes are associated with worse perceived pain, depression, and coping. Researchers at Cincinnati Children's Hospital took this a step further and investigated whether the tendency of parents to catastrophize influenced a child's coping and subsequent pain and functional limitations.[1] In their study, more than 70 percent of parent-child pairs coped similarly—parents who scored high on catastrophizing tended to have children high on catastrophizing. Even when controlling for parent pain history and severity of the child's pain in the past, parents who scored high on questionnaires about catastrophizing were likely to have children who reported similar attitudes. Additionally, children and parents who scored high in catastrophizing experienced more pain, more depression, and had lower levels of functioning.[2] The authors hypothesize that some of this may be genetic—an anxious parent may be prone to catastrophizing and anxiety is heritable.

However, another perspective is that parents with maladaptive coping skills can reinforce these on their children. Imagine a child who has had chronic pain has a day with moderate pain—if a parent tends to catastrophize, they may cancel the outing to the park to promote rest and begin medications, unintentionally teaching and reinforcing to the child that the pain is a limitation in their life. A parent with less catastrophic thinking may acknowledge the pain and work with the child to continue their planned activities while using whatever tools necessary for the child to be comfortable and cope with their pain. While it's frightening to parents to think that they have the potential to make a child's perceived pain and functioning worse by maladaptive coping, it's inspiring to think that if a parent learns healthier coping skills and models them for their child, they may be able to influence their child's well-being. This small study focused on pain management, but even if your child isn't coping with chronic pain, this evidence shows that it's possible for our attitudes to impact our children's health.

For this reason, one of the most helpful advanced parenting skills is bringing a positive, constructive mindset to your child's challenge. As parents, we have an opportunity to set the tone for our children and model the approach we would like them to take. While staying even-keeled amidst stress as a parent isn't easy, we'll discuss some strategies to help promote healthy coping.

"Growth mindset" is a term popularized by Carol Dweck, who describes it as follows in her bestselling book *Mindset*: "This growth mindset is based on the belief that your basic qualities are things you can cultivate through your efforts, your strategies, and help from others." The benefit of a growth mindset for typical children facing typical challenges is clear. It helps when you coach your child, saying, "You haven't mastered an academic skill *yet*, but by working hard you can accomplish your goals." Your child's state isn't static, and the growth mindset is founded in a belief in what's possible.

This approach can also help children who are not on a typical track: "You may have a big challenge dealing with your diagnosis, but I know with hard work and support from your doctors and teachers, you can learn to thrive with this." A growth mindset implies that the cards you are dealt are just a starting place and don't define your value. Your choices and actions have power.

For parents, similarly, when you face an unfamiliar or difficult task related to your child's challenge, a fixed mindset will have you feeling hopeless and thinking, "I can't do this." If you can work to adopt a growth mindset, the same challenge might spark you to say, "This is hard, but how can I learn to deal with this?" or, "Where can I get the help I need?" While difficult life experiences may train us to assume the worst and think catastrophically, we can learn and practice new productive responses that encourage a constructive growth mindset.

This is not to suggest that as a parent and caregiver you must possess limitless optimism and positivity. You will have your own reactions to this challenge, just as your child does. Parents who are anxious or who have a history of trauma may be particularly prone to imagining the worst. Additionally, we should give parents permission to experience big feelings in response to big stressors. It's okay to feel overwhelmed or down when facing something hard, but even in the hardest moments, remembering, "I can't do this *yet*," or "I haven't got a handle on how to deal with this *yet*," allows a parent to see that things can and likely will improve with time.

When you confront challenges as a parent, consider if the size of your feelings is in proportion to what's happening. Sometimes, a catastrophic feeling is there for good reason—perhaps there is an urgent concern that needs addressing. But other times, big feelings are there because your love for your child is so vast.

Why We Catastrophize—and How to Stop

As a parent, you are ultimately responsible when something goes wrong and the person most invested in your child's future. Many times, parent attention and vigilance makes a positive difference in a child's course. Parents have facilitated earlier diagnoses, recognized subtle signs, and even saved their children's lives. But, taken to the extreme, the benefit of increased vigilance and increased stress diminishes while the cost of excessive worries continues to accumulate. In an ideal scenario, we'd find a balance—a parent who is conscientious and responsive, but able to respond with intention and perspective rather than fear and anxiety.

If you tend toward catastrophic thinking, you can develop habits to break unwanted thought patterns and help you maintain perspective. These are some helpful steps that you can consider taking.

Triage

The Pareto principle is popularly referred to as the eighty-twenty rule. It estimates that 80 percent of the positive impact comes from 20 percent of the work. If there were a linear relationship between parenting work and child benefit, more effort would always result in better outcomes. But the eighty-twenty rule implies that 20 percent of our parenting work is responsible for 80 percent of the outcome. For parents facing challenges, some decisions are high stakes. Choosing the right surgery plan or the right doctors or the best school to support your child will have a profound impact and fall into the 20 percent category. Other decisions, like whether to ask for physical therapy once a week or twice a week, or whether to seek care on day one of a new illness or day three, will have a much less significant impact on your child's outcome. If you are someone who tends toward catastrophic thinking, it's likely that you will feel most decisions and situations are high in importance. But even though every decision that impacts your child may feel important, not everything is paramount in its effect. Pausing when you encounter a new symptom or a new problem to consider whether it's truly one of the important "game-changing" moments will help you to triage more effectively. Additional efforts and attention to the smaller decisions, while necessary and helpful, likely show fewer and fewer tangible benefits.

Compartmentalize

You can schedule a designated time for worrying each day, so that when troubling thoughts enter your mind you can remind yourself to set them aside to worry about later. This habit can allow you to practice letting thoughts "float by," rather than diving down a worry rabbit hole. It can free up emotional and mental bandwidth if you gently acknowledge the worry, and then remind yourself that you have dedicated time and space to process it later.

Reach Out to Friends and Family

We will talk in chapter 9 about maximizing your coping skills with positive self-talk, guided imagery, and humor, but spending time connecting with people you trust can be an invaluable way to gain support. Though it can be hard to find the right person—be it a friend, teacher, doctor, nurse, faith leader, or family member—they can provide essential support to help you understand your worries and to keep them in perspective. When you have someone to listen, venting about your stress can help, but be sure to be clear about your intention. Some parents seek support and reassurance, but their well-intended friends imagine they are looking for answers or logistic help. If you are seeking to vent worries but get ideas and solutions instead of the listening you want, you can end up feeling more overwhelmed. But if you ask for what you want up front—"I have a solid plan and still feel worried, would you just listen to what I'm dealing with?"—you may be more likely to get the support you need.

Find Professional Support

It's absolutely appropriate to mention feelings of anxiety to your child's care team. Sometimes pediatricians can change the care plan to enable more support. For example, when a pediatrician learns that a new mother is suffering from postpartum depression, our advice about feeding choices and mother's sleep may adjust to promote her coping. Similarly, if a family is struggling in coping with a challenge, we may be able to focus our advice more productively and more constructively. If a parent is struggling, it's not a good time to recommend a labor-intensive treatment. Not only would such a treatment add more stress, but it would also be less likely to be successful given the family dynamics. Sometimes we can connect families to others in similar circumstances or with support groups. Your care team can also help you decide if you need a therapist or psychiatrist for additional support of your mental health. For some parents, catastrophic thinking may be part of a larger underlying anxiety or a response to prior traumatic experiences, and sometimes addressing these bigger issues with professional help is the best course.

I worked with a parent whose son had survived lymphoma; as a result, she struggled with anxiety. Every time he had a sore throat or a sniffle, she would feel a swollen lymph node and imagine the cancer returning. When these worries were at their worst, she couldn't sleep or handle her daily activities like work and feeding her family. Even when he was well, she often had difficulty sleeping due to intrusive worries about his well-being. Her child's oncologist and I worked together to provide education and reassurance but encouraged her to seek additional mental health support to cope with her anxiety and catastrophic-thinking habits. She found a psychiatrist and took medication while she participated in cognitive behavioral therapy to learn and practice skills to cope with these intrusive and negative thoughts. While improvement did not come quickly or easily, this work helped her to take care of herself and her child.

Watching his mother engage in this work also showed the child, a tween at the time, that these resources could be of benefit. He ended up requesting to work with a therapist of his own to gain coping skills. While they still worried about his health, the subsequent spirals of worry tended to be hours instead of days or weeks, and the visits to see me became less frequent and the bags under the mother's eyes less dark.

Mind Your Own Health

In addition to affecting the tone of family life, catastrophic thinking can worsen the health of the parent. Remaining hypervigilant and chronically stressed will wear down your physical and emotional well-being. High stress reduces sleep quality and leads to a detrimental cycle of decreased coping capacity and worsening symptoms.

The stress response has an immediate and short-term effect on your body: to prepare for a crisis, your heart beats faster and harder, your breathing changes, and your hormones and glucose physiology adjust to increase your blood sugar. But long-term elevated stress also has significant consequences for your health, including increased rates of heart disease, cancer, diabetes, asthma, and depression.

It's no surprise that studies have shown that stress among caregivers can lead to their deteriorating health. An analysis of 547 studies of families with children affected by a variety of chronic physical conditions, such as asthma, cancer, cystic fibrosis, diabetes, epilepsy, juvenile rheumatoid arthritis, or sickle cell found that caregivers had significantly higher levels of stress than parents of children without health challenges.[3] The studies also showed that greater stress was associated with poorer mental resilience in caregivers *and* in children with chronic illness. The well-being of the parent is vital to the health of the children and the functioning of the family. Fortunately, there are steps that parents can take to reduce their stress and improve their well-being.

Where Are You Putting Your Energy?

I've had more than one parent threaten my life. This is not an unusual experience for my profession—many of my colleagues have reported receiving irrational threats. This happens so frequently that hospitals have protocols in place to protect doctors and nurses when necessary.

While I can't share much about how a specific situation escalates to this level, I can explain why. Sometimes a family is overwhelmed at their baseline—perhaps financially, socially, or due to other existing issues within the family—and now they face another crisis. A parent's emotions boil over and some feel the need to release those unbearable feelings. So, parents scream at the doctor, or they throw something at the nurse, or they curse at the receptionist and hang up.

These parents are not bad people. If you've done this before, you are not a bad person. Each time a parent has lashed out at me, it was because they were angry at the injustice of their child's situation and they were scared of losing their child. All those feelings erupted, and I was there. Even if you aren't the type to threaten a pediatrician, maybe there have been times when you lashed out at whoever happened to be there.

Other people respond to extreme stress in the opposite way—one-word answers, avoiding eye contact, not returning phone calls, and generally withdrawing. I once had a mother wear her sunglasses indoors for the duration of a visit. As I got to know her better, I saw this was her default; when she felt overwhelmed, uncertain, or untrusting, she would put up walls and plan to handle things on her own.

When you face a challenge, you have to put the energy of your reaction somewhere. Witnessing a family member's struggle is extraordinarily stressful. As you cope with that stress, where does it go? Parents often have a tendency toward either externalizing by taking the stress out on others or internalizing by taking the stress out on themselves. By understanding your tendencies, you can then choose to react more intentionally. Let's break down the two most common ways parents react in these difficult circumstances.

Externalizing—Taking Your Stress Out on Others

Parents who externalize may lash out angrily toward others. These individuals may get irritable and argumentative with team members. They may blame others when things don't go well. Externalizing has obvious costs, as alienating your doctor can reduce the quality of your care. In a less dramatic example, I know that if I walk in and the parent's arms are crossed and their answers are curt, then we won't have the open communication needed for good care.

Similarly, taking out your stress on teachers, therapists, or babysitters will carry a cost. Most of these people care for your child and won't retaliate, but if you damage the relationship, they will not have the smooth communication they need to provide your child with the best care. When the communication is open, your child's care team can learn about your goals, experiences, and home life, and this context can help them address your child's challenges more effectively.

While externalizing can be frustrating for your care team, most experienced providers can see that the families who are the angriest are often the ones that are suffering the most. If you catch yourself getting very angry, explain why. When your care team knows, they will be more equipped to offer the support you need.

Internalizing—Taking Your Stress Out on Yourself

If you internalize, you may blame yourself when things don't go well. You may feel hopeless or ashamed when you experience a setback. Parents who tend to internalize often experience stress and withdraw and isolate themselves. Some may even berate themselves. Understanding the consequences of this reaction may be more difficult for a parent to grasp at first.

Imagine a parent dealing with their child's eczema. They have followed the doctor's recommendations and administered medications, but the condition hasn't improved. Rather than confronting the doctor and communicating, "This isn't working and we need a new plan," the parent feels that something they did was wrong. They may do hours of research, purchase products recommended by sources they find online, and attempt to figure it out on their own. This reaction also comes at a cost. Speaking to the doctor or asking for help might have led to a better plan or would have helped the parent and child arrive at an answer more quickly.

Internalizing parents might assume that their struggles with getting their child's needs met is their fault, rather than the fault of a challenging condition or our byzantine health-care system. Furthermore, internalizing parents may be more likely to face health consequences, anxiety, or depression.[4] If you have a tendency to internalize, recognizing this can give you the opportunity to change your habits and reduce your risk of these complications.

Managing the Extremes

There are concerns with either extreme. By externalizing, you may drive away potential allies and miss opportunities for improvement. By internalizing, you may not voice your struggles sufficiently to get the support you need and your mental health may suffer. Whether you put too much blame on others or too much blame on yourself, you are likely to end up more isolated. And one of the most important things we can do to help families facing a challenge is to ensure they stay connected and avoid isolation.

The truth is, so many things are out of our control. We can't always prevent or predict the stress that we face, but we can control the way in which we respond. When presented with inevitable stress, if we can take a breath and broaden the gap, it can allow us to choose our own response. Psychologist Rollo May wrote about this in his article "Freedom and Responsibility Re-examined" in 1963: "Indeed I would define mental health as the capacity to be aware of the gap between stimulus and response, together with the capacity to use this gap constructively."[5]

You know yourself best. Whatever your go-to response might be, pause before you react. This may give you the opportunity to challenge yourself to intentionally change that response. If you are an externalizer and you are faced with an unexpected setback, you may need to say, "I need a minute." You can then take time to breathe deeply, or express your struggle to cope and need for help. This shift in response can prevent your taking your frustrations out on those around you, especially those who either didn't cause or cannot help the situation. If you tend to internalize, and you hit a wall regarding something your child needs, you may have to remind yourself to stay engaged and speak up to overcome the obstacle.

Working with Your Default Mode

We all have a default mode for how we handle stress. Antoine's father would withdraw like a turtle into his shell. Antoine had severe intellectual disability, self-injurious behavior, and epilepsy associated with a genetic syndrome. When he would experience a downturn—a worsening of his underlying diagnosis—Dad would seem to shrink, despite his over-six-foot frame. He would sort of nod along to the plan and subsequently wouldn't answer or return phone calls about Antoine's care for a few weeks.

I worried a lot about his family—whether they understood the complexity of his condition and whether they had enough help. But never for a moment did I doubt the father's dedication to his son. When he was ready, he would always be in touch to move forward with the plan. When his child needed immediate care, his father would always make it happen one way or another. As our relationship developed, instead of asking whether to move forward with this or that, I learned to ask, "Should we move forward now, or give you some time to process all this new information?" Antoine's dad would always elect more time. Often, we could work on his timeline more effectively than my own.

When Antoine was referred to see a new doctor, knowing that he moved a bit slower in making decisions and adapting to changes, I encouraged his father to speak up about his preferences for the timeline. Sometimes, physicians expect a rapid response, and a parent who doesn't move along to fill a new prescription or get blood work or testing right away might be labeled as "noncompliant" or even "negligent." If he wanted more time or more opportunity to learn about the decision at hand, communicating that would enable the new doctor to make a plan that better fit his preferences.

It's easy to label some of these instinctual reactions, particularly the ones that are at the extreme, as good or bad. However, just as we label all feelings valid, we should consider all responses acceptable. There is no right or wrong way to react when your child has a challenge—your reaction just *is*. Denying a problem, catastrophizing a symptom, taking your feelings out on others or yourself, are all valid ways that parents try to cope. I'd encourage you to give grace to yourself as you think about how you and your family members fit into these patterns. The point isn't to change your default response or to change your responses to fit those expected by your care team. Simply knowing and understanding your default response can empower you. Once you see your tendency and name it, you allow yourself agency. You can choose the best way to proceed and make a plan to help yourself and your child. In this way, awareness and knowledge are power.

Before you move on, consider the following questions:

- What are you bringing to your child's experience?
- Are there any strengths you bring to the situation you haven't considered?
- What are your limitations and where are your blind spots?
- Is your reaction the right size for what you face?
- Are you one to internalize or externalize stress?

CHAPTER 2

What Matters Most?

When I was first diagnosed with cancer at age four, my parents tearfully sat me down. They explained my diagnosis and told me a bit about what would come: procedures, chemotherapy, and radiation. But as a four-year-old, only one thing mattered to me. Amidst this very serious and stressful conversation, I grew wide-eyed and asked, "But I can still play, right?"

To understand how a challenge will affect your child, you first have to understand where they are and what matters to them most. For my family, as I was going through the appointments, surgeries, and chemo schedule, prioritizing my play was paramount. They knew the open hours for the hospital playroom and used toy-store trips strategically to bribe me through painful or unpleasant parts of my challenge.

However, my needs were just one part of the family needs. My mom had just signed up to go to school at night on top of her full-time job. My dad was living a few hours away to take advantage of a job opportunity that meant increased income for my family. We didn't have family nearby who would help take care of me, so they had to make decisions about what would give and what wouldn't. My mom wanted to try to make her plan to study for her MBA at night work, because in the long run it would be good for all of us.

Understanding all the perspectives and needs of your household can feel like peeling back layers of an onion. Sometimes you may need to be clear and selective about what your priorities are so that you can make necessary choices. Most parents instinctively keep their child's priorities centered to anchor their thought processes.

But to make the best choices, you have to balance your child's needs with those of the broader family too—the parents, the siblings, and any other household members. Every family has multiple balls in the air. Some are bouncy balls and if you drop them the show will go on. But others are glass and require more attention to keep intact.

Some of these particularly tough choices have difficult but necessary solutions. I've worked with countless families who had to make hard decisions around a parent's job. In one case, the mother of one of my patients could not stay with her daughter in the hospital because if she missed more work, she would lose her job, and if she lost her job, she'd lose the family health insurance.

But outside of these obvious, important, urgent priorities, there is a whole spectrum of other priorities. Some for you, some for your co-parent, some for your children, some for your work, friends, or other family members. As you consider all your needs and which are your priorities, I'd encourage you use this simple Eisenhower decision matrix[1] as a guide.

	Urgent	Not Urgent
Important		
Not Important		

In the Eisenhower Matrix, important and urgent priorities go in one quadrant. These are the front-burner items like your child being sick and requiring a hospital visit. Not important but urgent priorities may include things like grocery shopping, doing laundry, and ensuring child-care for other children. These have to get done but can sometimes be delegated. Important, not urgent work may include longer-term projects like deciding which school to attend, researching a medical condition, or hiring help. Nonurgent and unimportant tasks are ones we're probably already minimizing.

Most people address urgent important priorities first because they identify the glass ball. But when we have more on our plate, we can forget the important nonurgent goals. A parent who has been feeling overwhelmed has decided it is important to hire more help, but since it's not urgent, a few weeks go by before they begin the process to obtain that help. Another family has been juggling two children with acute needs and was counting on their third low-maintenance child to get by more independently. But over time this child begins to have emotional difficulties and seeks support from potentially troubling sources.

Some of these important, nonurgent needs can and should wait while you are dealing with something more pressing, but the important needs like long-term goals and attending to the more stable sibling should eventually get attention. By remembering what your priorities are, you can redirect your energy toward addressing what matters most.

We should minimize spending time and energy attending to not important and not urgent priorities whenever possible. Identifying what fits in this box can be elusive; many people might say "social media" or "phone time," but sometimes the point of those activities is to connect with others, to do research, or to relax and decompress—things that may be priorities.

Now, take a few minutes to imagine your child's matrix. While it may seem like a silly exercise depending on the age and stage of your child, children do have their own priorities. My priority was to play. Many toddlers will demand to be free to explore their environment, many children have a deep and important need to spend time with their closest friend, and many teens have a pressing need for privacy and independence. While their health is essential, one of your most important jobs as a parent is to help your child identify and protect their priorities.

Here are two samples of what this matrix might look like. Let's imagine that Sam is an eight-year-old boy with type 1 diabetes.

Child's priorities

	Urgent	Not Urgent
Important	Protecting time to play baseball Asserting independence	Relationships with friends Feeling good
Not important	Eating, sleeping Minimizing disruptions to school Not feeling "weird"	Long-term goals like acquiring a new skill or preventing a complica- tion from diabetes.

Parent's priorities for child

	Urgent	Not Urgent
Important	Optimizing safety Promoting wellness, health, and academic skills	Relationships with parents and siblings
Not important	Eating, sleeping, hygiene Appropriate supplies and childcare	Relationships with friends Playing baseball

What you might see here is that both the parent and the child share some priorities—eating, sleeping, and relationships are on the radar and appear on both matrixes. But Sam will see some things like friendship and baseball as much more important and much more urgent than his parents. Because his frontal cortex—the area of the brain that helps him make decisions—is still developing, it is quite normal that he would not prioritize thinking about his safety or long-term control of diabetes.

In your home, each family member may have their unique perspectives and priorities—and none are necessarily right or wrong. But when you compare each family member's matrix, you will see some areas where priorities align well and other areas where priorities differ or are in tension. If you, as the primary caregiver, power through acting on your priorities, ignoring these tensions, your connection with other stakeholders in your home may suffer because they don't share the goal.

Some parents might say, "He is just a kid; I have way too much on my plate to worry about baseball too." And in the short-term that decision may be the perfect choice for your family—for whatever financial or logistic considerations you may face. But in the long run, if over and over you choose based on your priority grid without acknowledging the goals of your co-parent or child, they may feel their priorities and preferences aren't heard and your relationship may suffer.

Mindfulness about all the different priorities can help you be more thoughtful about the balance you choose. In the next sections, we'll break down some of the most common needs for children and adults and talk about how we can best support our children and ourselves as we establish priorities. While there are a lot of needs to consider, we can't possibly prioritize all of them all the time.

Universal Needs

Jasleen was a two-and-a-half-year-old girl who was born preterm and had some developmental delays. She was small, but very feisty and active. The most significant issue was her swallowing skills; due to a suspected neurological injury, she was unable to swallow thin liquids and used a feeding tube to maintain hydration. Her feedings had to be carefully conducted, as unfortunately if the feeds went in too quickly, she suffered reflux and would have pain or spit-up.

Jasleen's parents brought her to my office to address her reflux, but the real issue was helping the family select their priorities. She attended physical therapy, occupational therapy, speech therapy, and feeding therapy, and was making meaningful progress in all of them. While advancing her intake so that she could eat and drink without the feeding tube was an important, nonurgent goal, the feeding therapy was over an hour-long drive away from their home. Between all this and school there wasn't enough time to feed her.

The family had considered various ways to adjust her schedule issues, but none of the options seemed to work for them. If she got the hydration by feeding tube while she was sleeping, it would be bad for her reflux;

while in the car she might get carsick; right before physical therapy she might be uncomfortable. Outside of taking her to her appointments, the mom had to do laundry, cook, and take care of another child. And Jasleen also needed free play time to practice all her hard-earned skills, and to just be a kid. To make it fit, something had to give.

As I tried to solve this scheduling issue, the discussion of all the family's needs became necessary. These human truths are too often neglected in a doctor's office, but when doctors are making a medical plan, recognizing basic universal needs is essential.

Parents and children have some predictable needs. All of us need rest, movement, time outdoors, sustenance, consistency, and love. While these may sound obvious, I see these needs neglected all the time both for caregiving parents and their children. I'll review each of these needs here and make an argument for why they should continue to be a priority for you moving forward. As you read, consider which universal needs you have been neglecting, and consider if there's a way to give them the attention they deserve.

Rest

The science is very clear here: few things are as essential to well-being as sleep. Sleep helps with behavior, mood, healing, immunity, learning, and growth. Yet, our institutions—hospitals, schools, workplaces, day cares—do not seem to prioritize child or parent sleep.

A school with services better suited to your child might require a longer drive and earlier wake-up time. A physical therapist might only have availability during your child's typical nap time. The doctor prescribed the medication to be taken four times a day and you can't seem to get the doses in during your child's twelve waking hours.

Most parents observe the consequences of insufficient child sleep. We know that sleep-deprived children have more behavior problems and more difficulty regulating their emotions. Additionally, in academic settings, sleep-deprived children demonstrate decreased memory, worse cognitive performance, and are less alert.[2] Sleep deprivation has also been shown to impair children's growth.[3]

Generally, getting a child to sleep is one of the hardest and most complex parts of parenting. When a child faces a challenge, sometimes sleep can become even more difficult. A child may have symptoms that interrupt sleep—like a child with eczema who wakes up scratching themselves, or a child with asthma who wakes when coughing. A child may have medical needs that interrupt sleep; for instance when a child with diabetes needs to have their blood sugar checked in the middle of the night, or children who need late-night feeds or medication. Setting limits and managing sleep hygiene issues like screen time is a challenge for all children, but when you add behavioral challenges or mental health stressors it can be even harder.

I would recommend that parents focus on the things they can control. Keeping sleep as a priority will lead you to make better choices about the daily schedule, bedtime routine, screen time, and other sleep-hygiene issues. When you are facing your child's sleep challenges, make sure you ask your care team for help and tailored advice to support your sleeping goals. As the parent, you may often need to push your care team and say things like, "I understand you want me to do this in the morning, but this would mean waking up too early to be sustainable. Are there other options?"

Disrupted children's sleep leads to reduced sleep for parents. In addition to supporting our children at night, parents often end up staying up nights to do additional caregiver work, including medical research, organization, and ordering health products. Or because we were so busy attending to these tasks during the day, the only time we have for ourselves is in the evening after the children go to bed.

When your sleep as a caregiver is inadequate or interrupted, your health and well-being will suffer too. A recent analysis of several studies found that sleep disruption was one of the most common physical health risks reported by caregivers.[4] Regular poor sleep puts you at risk for serious medical conditions, including depression,[5] coronary heart disease,[6] and diabetes.[7] It shortens your life expectancy by as much as 15 percent.[8] Consistent lack of sleep can put you at more risk for getting infections.[9] Sleep deprivation slows your response time and may have safety implications when it comes to driving.[10]

The most concerning aspect of this is that building a sleep debt impairs your ability to cope, which can subsequently lead to a cycle of worsening overall functioning.[11] Chronic sleep deprivation decreases your ability to make good decisions. Dealing with the consequences of poor decisions leads to more stress. More stress makes everything worse and leads to more sleep deprivation. Sleep-deprived caregivers are less capable of the work that drove them to become sleep deprived.

Being proactive and protective about sleep is essential. However, as you've probably been thinking while reading this section, getting adequate sleep for many feels impossible, particularly if you have urgent, important demands in the middle of the night. I've worked with parents who were working nights and watching their kids all day and squeezing in rest when they could, and some of these decisions between bad (having a job and feeling terrible all the time) and worse (quitting your job and facing homelessness) reflect some of our societal dysfunction. Some of these burdens can feel impossible to solve at the individual level.

However, despite these barriers, there are things that we can do to help. First is to know that you are not alone in working to promote your child's sleep and your own. If you speak up about needing help promoting and protecting sleep, you should be able to get support. Many parents assume the sleep piece is just something they have to figure out on their own, but precisely because sleep is so important for your child and for you, your care team should prioritize it.

In some situations, a child may have real medical needs that interrupt sleep that can't be rescheduled. Taking turns on nighttime care with a co-parent, family member, or babysitter can help you prevent the sleep problems from falling consistently on one person. It's common for families to prioritize the sleep of the parent who may be doing paid work over caregiving work during the day. While sometimes this makes sense, unless the caregiver is allowed an opportunity for rest during the day—when another caregiver is present or perhaps when the child goes to school—it's unfair.

Sometimes, the published ideals feel out of reach, but even small changes can add up to make a big difference. You can set an alarm to remind yourself to go to bed earlier, or you can block off time during the day for a brief nap. You can restrict your screen time right before bed or use a white-noise machine or black-out curtains to improve your sleep environment. Focusing on your own sleep hygiene can help improve the quality of your sleep, even if you can't significantly increase the amount of sleep. Remember also that there are seasons of parenting and habits evolve as children grow. In some seasons your sleep may be a lower priority, and that's okay too.

Movement

Physical activity and sleep are variables that are difficult to isolate—well-rested individuals tend to be more energetic and active, and individuals who are active tend to have improved sleep quality and quantity.

We have strong evidence that in adults, physical activity reduces risk of coronary heart disease, high blood pressure, stroke, metabolic syndrome, type 2 diabetes, breast and colon cancer, depression, and falls. Put another way, physical inactivity, defined as having less than twenty minutes of moderate physical activity a day, or less than ten minutes of vigorous physical activity a day, is a major health risk. Physical inactivity has been described as the fourth leading cause of death—over five million theoretically preventable deaths a year are ascribed to physical inactivity. Yet inactivity remains common, with nearly 31 percent of the world not meeting recommendations.[12]

For most children, much of the school day is sedentary. Some schools are becoming more mindful of prioritizing physical activity, as it's shown to improve learning, but this has yet to be reliably and nationally prioritized in public education. Families also might struggle to help their children stay active, as there can be logistical, transportation, and cost hurdles when it comes to signing kids up for sports or dance classes.

For children with disabilities, it can be nearly impossible to find appropriate resources to promote physical activity. Hippotherapy, a type of language and occupational therapy using horses, can do wonders for children with cerebral palsy, sensory needs, and autism, but the cost can be prohibitive and not all parts of the country have horses. Finding a swim lesson for a child with a typical developmental trajectory is often challenging. There are few pools and many children, but when you add in a challenge such as cerebral palsy or needing wheelchair access, it can be impossible to find an accessible swim class. Increasing access is not just important ethically, but also medically—the benefits of the sensory experience of time in the water and the gravity-free exercise can be invaluable for disabled children in reducing pain, improving sleep, and helping promote appetite and digestion.

While the barriers can be considerable, the benefits of movement are so great that it's worth devoting time to overcoming them. Movement centers one's mood and improves cognition, behavior, appetite, bowel movements, immune response, and cardiovascular fitness. When I help families find ways to promote their child's movement, I often focus on the schedule and structure of the day. While some young children will find a way to be vigorously active in a room alone with a cardboard box, for other children physical activity needs to be planned and facilitated. In addition to scheduling, the following tips can help you incorporate more physical activity into your child's day:

- **Trial and error:** Don't give up if the first attempt at dance or sports doesn't interest your child. It's worthwhile to invest time in finding an activity your child enjoys.
- **Make it fun:** Many adults approach exercise as a chore, but when we find ways to make physical activity fun for all involved—games, competition, sports, exploration, or imaginary play—it facilitates more frequent activity by promoting intrinsic motivation.

- **Physical activity with family and friends:** Many children exercise more intently and for longer duration when it's also a social activity. If you enjoy walking, jogging, or biking, find a way to include your children. Should this fail, try to include their peers. My children will complain or feel bored on a hike with me, but when their friends come along, they enjoy the activity more and have more endurance.
- **School selection:** When I was picking a school for my children, I noticed that some schools devoted zero resources to movement, while others spent up to an hour and a half encouraging children to move as part of the school day. When considering a school, weigh this among the deciding factors.
- **School partnerships:** If your child has difficulties with school or an individualized education plan (IEP) to provide accommodations, you can make plans to utilize movement as a coping skill (if my child is upset or having trouble focusing, he will be allowed to go for a walk or stand at his desk). And parents and educators should be mindful never to punish children by taking away their favored movement activity, such as a child with behavioral difficulties associated with ADHD who is restricted from recess. Decreasing a child's opportunity to move will almost certainly worsen behavior, and movement is so essential, in some ways this would be similar to restricting access to food or sleep.

Caregivers may also struggle to find time in the day to exercise. Just like for children, exercise takes time, energy, space, and often money. It can be essential to find activities you can do on your terms, in your own space or neighborhood. Some parents may find that it helps to change their perspective on exercise, from considering it an optional luxury to prioritizing it as a central necessity. Most parents don't forget to brush their teeth, and once a habit has had enough repetition built in, it can become routine.

Personally, I found the most successful strategy to promote more exercise is mindfulness. During the pandemic, when my mental health was not in a good place, exercise provided me with a boost in mood, enhanced focus, and renewed energy. A mindful moment to check in with myself before and after exercise allowed me to observe the lift in my mood and energy level. Now, whenever I feel like I don't have the time to exercise, I remind myself of how tangible those benefits have been, mentally and physically. While I know there are long-term health benefits to exercise, the direct and immediate benefits are much more motivating to me. I know that feeling better and functioning better after exercise is well worth the trouble.

Time Outdoors and Nature

Another priority frequently forgotten is time connecting with nature. We know that in nature, the sights, sounds, and smells activate our parasympathetic nervous system in a way that directly reduces the cortisol-induced "fight or flight" side of our nervous system. Exposure to bright light, especially in the morning, can promote healthy sleep by regulating our circadian rhythm and melatonin secretion. For children, as little as an hour outdoors daily has been shown to reduce the risk of myopia, or nearsightedness.[13]

Studies have shown that time in green spaces improves physical activity and blood pressure, promotes cognitive skills, and reduces potential for anxiety and depression.[14] In her book *The Nature Fix*, Florence Williams describes the prolific research showing how powerfully beneficial time outdoors is for our health, something that's embraced in other parts of the world, but deemphasized by some Western cultures.

Most parents do not have time outdoors on their radar as a priority. While finding a safe, comfortable way to spend time outdoors amidst your other commitments may be difficult, I suspect you'll find the mental and physical health benefits well worth the effort. For inspiration, the organization 1000 Hours Outside seeks to encourage matching screen time with time outdoors. You can accomplish this goal by leaving a chunk of time on the weekend for an outdoor outing or by adding smaller chunks of outdoor time regularly, such as adding fifteen minutes to an errand to visit a park nearby.

Sustenance

Parents intuitively focus on their child's nutrition. Feeding your offspring is a deeply held instinct, so this is not a need that a parent is likely to neglect. Sometimes though, when your child's nutrition is part of their challenge, it can become medicalized. The need to quantify and the pressure to optimize each meal can be overwhelming and begin to box out the joy and pleasure of a shared meal. As you consider your priorities, please remember that feeding is more than calories and nutrients in. For our children and ourselves, food should be restorative; it should be an opportunity for enjoyment, and a touchstone for connection and community.

While parents nearly never forget to feed a child, most parents have skipped meals. Our children's needs tend to come before our own, and it seems a small sacrifice to make. However, we know that adequate nutrition is essential to fuel good health. The health consequences of skipping meals have been studied in adolescents, in whom skipping breakfast has been shown to lead to worse school performance, increased psychosocial difficulties, and decreased dietary quality, specifically less fruit and fewer foods dense in vitamin D, calcium, and iron.[15] We can assume for caregiving parents, similarly when a meal is skipped, those calories are still consumed in the form of snacks, which generally have lower nutrient density.

Amidst the chaos of a challenge, it's easy to let the structure of your day slide, but regular meals, just like regular sleep, are an important part of keeping your energy up and your health intact so you can support your family's needs. Increasingly, the nascent field of nutritional psychiatry recognizes the impact of foods on mental health due to the neurological connections between the gut and the brain. In her book *This Is Your Brain on Food,* psychiatrist Uma Naidoo explores the science of how traditional comfort foods high in sugar and on the glycemic index may actually worsen symptoms of depression, and how the traditional Western diet may lead to excess anxiety through negatively impacting the microbiome. Other foods high in fiber, vitamin D, magnesium or healthy bacteria are thought to help.

If you struggle to find time to feed yourself, I encourage you to ask for help. While you may not be able to delegate or outsource some aspects of the challenge, nutrition is one area where you may find people willing and able to help. Planning ahead can also lighten your load—making lunch at breakfast time or batch cooking four days of lunch one evening.

Consistency

Routines can make us feel safe in a way that words cannot. Children are resilient and can adapt to all sorts of scenarios when it's necessary, but knowing what's coming next helps them feel safe.

One of the families I worked with had five kids, all of whom ended up in the hospital at one time or another due to chronic medical conditions. When I asked how the children coped so well, the parents pointed to their dedication to providing caregiving consistency. When one of their children was in the hospital for months, they tapped a network of people to help with logistics and meals. With this support in place, one parent always stayed at the hospital overnight and one parent was always at home overnight. Weeks went by when the parents were like ships passing in the night, but their young children, while worried about their sibling's health, took great comfort in their ability to count on the predictability of a present parent.

When you face a challenge, disruptions to the routine are inevitable. Unexpected errands, appointments, and illnesses occur, but you can keep your routines consistent. A predictable scaffolding will increase your children's cooperation with the routine and decrease power struggles.

Routines are established best practices at improving mealtimes and bed-times for children. Evidence suggests that for children facing a challenge such as type 1 diabetes, cystic fibrosis, or treatment for cancer, routines can promote parent and child well-being, as well as treatment adherence although routines can be difficult to implement successfully.[16–18] For the caregiving parent, a routine can allow you to have protected time for the work that you need to do or for yourself. A predictable routine can also help reduce the number of decisions you make in a day and conserve mental energy.

While some people gain a sense of control from a well-organized cal-endar, a routine can be much simpler and entail a portion of your day that becomes familiar and automatic. When you have a routine in place, such as homework followed by dinner, a shower, and quiet reading time, your child will feel safe and seen, even if you're not immediately avail-able as a parent.

Love

All people need love, and to feel heard and seen. Safe, stable, nurtur-ing relationships have been found to promote positive health outcomes across the life span by mitigating the impact of toxic stress.[19] Unfortu-nately, facing a challenge can be inherently isolating for children and their caregiving parents.

Establishing positive social relationships is a complex skill relying on emotional regulation, empathy, and communication skills. Many chil-dren need help acquiring these skills. Sometimes it is necessary to pri-oritize these skills over other academic or milestone skills, as emotional skills can facilitate a child's other abilities and may reap substantial ben-efits for a child's overall functioning and happiness. Sometimes parents try to meet a child's social needs within the family unit and may be hesi-tant or skeptical to ask for outside assistance with this aspect.

When it comes to friends and social supports, even a few meaningful connections outside the household can provide valuable complementary perspectives. The relationship a parent has with a child is special, but parents are not the only ones who can provide love and connection. Extended family members, teachers, paid caregivers, friends, and all sorts of people from their community can do so as well.

To meet your child's need for love:

- Leave time in the schedule for you and your child to connect in a positive way—such as reading, cuddling, or playing.
- Teach your child the skills to build and maintain important relationships and facilitate their friendships.
- View other adults who provide your child with unconditional love and support as treasured resources for your child.
- Model prioritizing relationships in your own life.

Many parents view investing time in friendships as a luxury, but in truth these relationships can be invaluable resources to promote coping and happiness, and to provide respite, support, and understanding. But friendships do take time and energy, and as with any relationship there are boundaries to maintain. When you bring these people into your life and your household, you model for your children these important skills.

The friends you had prior to becoming a parent, or prior to becoming a parent who is facing a challenge, might not carry over through all seasons in your life. Often this is because these friends lack knowledge and experience to empathize with what you are dealing with. We'll talk more about harnessing the good in your relationships in Chapters 7 and 10.

Safety

Some challenges directly threaten our child's safety and rise to the top of our priority list. Everyone needs to feel safe, including caregivers, siblings, and other household members. If a child has a life-threatening medical issue, it can be nearly as important for the child to *feel* safe, as it is for them to actually be safe. Many may find the experience of being diagnosed with a life-threatening condition to be a traumatic event in itself, and some will require time to process and recover from this news.

When doctors address families facing food allergies, asthma, or epilepsy, they have to emphasize how essential being prepared and vigilant is to the child's health. But doctors and caregivers need to choose their words carefully for communicating in front of and with that child. The conversation needs to be framed in an empowering tone. Striking a balance is a challenge, but an important one. I'll talk more about how to adjust your communication style to meet your child's developmental status in Chapter 8.

You may have picked up this book looking to make things easier, not to be reminded of all the needs your family has, which may feel like more to-dos than you can handle. But frequently families facing challenges are destabilized and thrown off course by what they face. In the introduction, I mentioned a family friend whose child had a recent diagnosis of asthma due to recurrent wheezing with viral illnesses. The family had a big scare, and several emergency-room visits for breathing concerns. But amidst the chaos of parenting two kids and worrying that one may struggle to breathe in the middle of the night, my friend had lost her bearings. She hadn't slept well in weeks. She had given up on maintaining a bedtime routine and both of her children weren't sleeping well either. She was indecisive, irritable, and not herself.

For her and for so many of the families I have worked with, prioritizing these basic self-care practices—rest, movement, time outdoors, sustenance, consistency, and love—is the first step to improving caregiving. She was inherently capable of learning about this new diagnosis and making and enacting a plan for her children, but until she got the rest she needed to function appropriately, she would feel adrift and overwhelmed. These universal needs are essential to prioritize as part of your caregiving plan for your family. Next, we'll move on to discuss the unique needs of your family and how to balance conflicting priorities, but before we do, take a moment to consider:

- Which needs are most essential to your child now?
- Which needs are most essential for you now?
- What needs have you done a good job prioritizing?
- Which needs have been neglected recently?

Unique Needs

Every now and then in my practice I've gotten to see glimpses of my patients' lives outside of the clinic. I've learned that the adolescent with cerebral palsy also has an enormous passion for trains and maintains a YouTube channel. The eight-year-old girl with diabetes is devoted to spending hours a day dancing. The siblings with sickle cell are also markedly accomplished in their sports and schoolwork.

At the center of all this is a child—your child. In an ideal world, your family, your caregiving support team, your medical or educational team—everyone would be rallied around supporting the child. This means instead of fitting the child into the protocol, you adapt the protocol to fit the needs of the child.

Designing a plan in this way may seem obvious, as of course that's how parents make decisions for their children. But medical and educational systems were not designed in this way. As these systems improve, slowly but surely, they will become more family centered and child centered. But in reality, parents still have to advocate to ensure their family's values and needs are at the center of the decisions made for their child.

This is not always easy given the power dynamic parents experience in many of these settings. The doctors and educators you encounter may have credentials or experience that will guide their plans for your child. Some people may find this dynamic intimidating. However, your expertise on your child and your family is equally if not more valuable for making plans for your child. Please don't be afraid to speak up when you feel your child is being asked to conform to a protocol, rather than vice versa.

While you know what excites and delights your child and what your child detests, the only individual who is more of an authority on your child is your child. When you are approaching decisions about your child, you should consider what your child would choose if it were up to them. This is an important practice, even if they are too young or developmentally unable to participate in the decision-making process.

In many scenarios, considering your child's preference will not impact your decision. As parents, we know when our toddler needs to take an essential medication, even if they do not want to. We're the ones who will help them make the right choice. But there are increasingly large gray zones where we could just decide, or we could respect the child's decision-making. We'll talk more about navigating the tension between your preferences and your child's preferences in Chapter 8. But as you consider your priorities, push yourself to also consider those of your child.

- What is your child's number-one priority?
- Does your care team know what matters most to your child?
- If your child were in charge of the plan, what would be different?
- What's one way you could adapt your plan to be more centered around your child?

When the Needs Are Overwhelming

With your child facing a challenge, there will be additional needs that require your time and energy as a caregiver. Parents will need to manage research, care coordination, additional childcare, and emergency planning. These tasks often require substantial time, intellect, and energy. Unfortunately, this work is unpaid and often goes unnoticed, but is essential to the well-being of your child and your family. We'll talk more about how to cope with the emotions around these new responsibilities in Chapter 9 and about how to create a plan that is sustainable in Chapter 12. But for now, the most important thing to note is that you need to make room for these responsibilities while balancing all of the other needs.

Parents need to understand the universal and evolving needs of family members and children. But this logistical work can also be emotional and overwhelming. In primary care, I work with parents to meet the universal needs of every child for rest, movement, time outdoors, sustenance, consistency, and love. By the end of our discussion, I can see that parents are overwhelmed by it all—and these are parents of relatively healthy children. As a caregiver, you face additional needs.

If you're feeling overloaded, I urge you to zoom out a little. As you think about all of these needs, understand it's less important to meet every need every day as perfectly as possible. One meal is never a good proxy to know if you have a healthy diet; within every diet, some meals are higher in protein and others higher in fiber, some with more added sugar and some with excess fats. When we think of nutrition, we think of our diets over a week or a month or a year.

In the same vein, there may be seasons of your parenting journey where everyone gets a lot of physical activity or no one gets any sleep. There may be times when you are very connected with your co-parent or very disconnected with your child, and that's okay. We aren't aiming to score 100 percent, as this is life, not a test.

Choosing which needs to deprioritize is one of the most difficult tasks of caregiving. Often, like with Jasleen, I see doctors recommended a lot of developmental therapies for a preschool child experiencing some delays. If a child is in preschool half the day, and regularly napping, and encouraged to have physical, occupational, and speech therapy, there may be little time or energy left for anything else. Your schedule may get to a place where you have to draw the line. You might decide that even though daily therapy might be more beneficial than three times a week, you have to leave time for play, rest, and connection. In situations like these, you make the best decision you can and go from there.

Aligning Priorities Among Stakeholders

There are, of course, other opinions involved. Your co-parent, other family members, health-care professionals, or paid caregivers may have strong opinions about how you define your priorities. We all bring our own values to parenting. In real life, it may take substantial negotiation to get everyone on the same page, but the time and energy devoted to this will often make things easier down the line. Furthermore, having the same plan can potentially avoid disagreements and disappointments.

Jason is a seven-year-old boy who is shy and tentative. He has had difficulty making and maintaining friendships. He is a worrier and often has difficulty sleeping. He asks for a lot of reassurance and sometimes avoids activities he labels as challenging or scary. He has strong preferences about the clothing he wears because of texture sensitivities. You can imagine that his parents may have different opinions about whether and when to seek help for Jason. Some of these opinions will be influenced by facts. The parent who spends more time with the child—who directly observes him struggling, answers calls from the school, or answers his calls for reassurance—may be the one to suggest he get an evaluation about anxiety. If the other parent doesn't know because of inadequate communication, they may disagree.

Or one parent may view these characteristics as part of Jason's inborn personality, as he has always been this way. This parent may feel that a psychologist would be going too far, and that it'd be better to just arrange more after-school activities and playdates to pull Jason out of his shell. This parent may feel that there are other family issues that are more pressing for them to address first.

The other parent may feel that time invested in therapy to improve Jason's coping and self-regulation skills will enable him to make progress with friendships. This may be their top priority over the other family needs.

This disagreement may get heated, and so the first step would be to de-escalate the conflict. The parents may find that identifying the discrepancy as one related to priorities rather than values can be a helpful step. If the priority is first for me and third for my partner, I can understand why he has other pressing matters to attend to, but at least it's on his list. If my priority is not on his list, I begin to worry that we don't see things the same way and that our disagreement represents a deeper rift in our relationship. When you care so deeply about the topic at hand—your child's well-being—this can feel very upsetting and personal. Family members want to share important beliefs and values, and often they want to align in love and devotion to their children.

In this scenario, Jason's parents both see he is struggling and want to solve the problem in different ways. If a disagreement is about the best time and method to achieve their shared goal, that feels manageable. But deeper arguments about decisions based on distinct beliefs and values can be much more difficult to navigate. The parent who is hesitant to pursue therapy may view Jason's tendencies as part of who he is and be offended at the suggestion of "changing him." Or the parent may believe that therapy is ineffective, or that it's the role of the parent to address issues like these.

These beliefs may evoke strong reactions, and I imagine you can guess which parent I might side with in this disagreement. Conversations about these beliefs may be emotionally charged, but it will be very difficult to proceed to do what's best for Jason without first getting on the same page. Once you know why your co-parent doesn't want to proceed with therapy, you can discuss those deeper beliefs and find resources to find common ground or steps forward. One parent could suggest that they both have a consultation with a therapist before committing to therapy, so that the hesitant parent can ask questions without feeling the need to commit right away. This can also open up time for the hesitant parent to learn more about the advantages of pursuing evaluation and treatment.

Naming, knowing, and agreeing to these priorities as a family will help parents to better advocate for their child. When both parents have their priorities in place, they can share them with the whole care team to help everyone reach shared goals.

So now, take a moment to consider where you, your co-parent, and your family members are when it comes to your values and priorities:

- What are your priorities?
- Are there conflicting priorities within your family?
- What are constructive ways you can help everyone agree to your child's care plan?

Getting the Professionals on the Same Page

In the 1960s, my uncle was diagnosed with cancer when he was two years old. His parents were allowed to visit an hour a day and weren't given many details or allowed much input about his care. During this time, families were tolerated rather than respected. By the time I had cancer in 1987, things were different. Pediatricians and hospitals then understood that unnecessary separation of children from their parents could be traumatic, and they had begun to make a habit of including parents in care decisions.

The same year I got sick, Surgeon General C. Everett Koop's public-health campaign centered on empowering families. Koop's closing remarks at the 1987 Surgeon General's Conference asked for "the development of systems of care at the community level that demonstrate responsiveness to the strengths and needs of families, that are developed through partnership between parents and professionals."[20]

Today, while we haven't necessarily made family-centered care a reality, it's squarely acknowledged as a priority and best practice in medicine. At the core of this family-centered movement is a respect for what matters most to families. Rather than apply a one-size-fits-all approach to making medical decisions, we now incorporate a family's beliefs and preferences to make the best plan.

In practice, this means it's common to delay a procedure that may impact summer swimming lessons or to discharge a child at a time of day that works best for the parents' work schedules or siblings' school schedules. In order to do this well, the medical team needs parents to share information about the family's needs. When I was starting my complex-care practice, one of the most important pieces of advice I received was to not focus so much on the bad days that I forget to ask about the patients' good days.

Sharing your child's passions and family priorities with your team, medical and otherwise, will help them respect what's important to you. Sometimes rushed appointments don't leave much time or opportunity for connecting at this level. It's important that you feel seen and understood by your doctor, so that may mean interrupting and saying something along the lines of, "Before we move on, I want to emphasize that my priority for this visit is improving my child's sleep, because we can't continue to function like this." What matters to your child should matter to everyone on the team, but if they don't see what you see as a parent, they won't know how to support your child's passions.

It may be surprising, but even though it seems like your child's medical team is focused on procedures, medications, and lab work, they also care about supporting your child's hobbies, athletic interests, and friendships. This represents a fundamental shift in the way we think of medical care. All parents advocate for their children, but caregiving parents must take those extra steps to ensure the team is aligned in a broader sense. Caregivers face higher stakes and more complex decisions, which is why communicating what's important to your child and your family is so essential. But before you can tackle communicating with others, identifying and aligning your family's priorities in the context of your unique situation is a valuable step.

As you move forward, coming back to what's most important will help ground you. In the next chapter, we'll dive into a landscape analysis of the common medical and educational resources. While many families know about these different pieces of care, thinking critically about how we use each resource can help support your efforts to support your family through a challenge. Before we dive into these details, reflect on what matters most to your family:

- What's most important to your child now, in the short-term?
- Are there areas where you have been neglecting your own needs to the detriment of your wellness?
- What passions do you want to prioritize for yourself and your family in the long-term?

CHAPTER 3

Medical and Educational Literacy

Some people seem to sail through life even when they face hardship, while others seem destined to have a much harder time. Socioeconomic status, race, ethnicity, sexual orientation, sex, disability, geographic location, and educational attainment are widely understood to be social determinants of health and predictors of which individuals have an easier time facing challenges. Social determinants of health have a profound effect on health outcomes.[1] Examples of this are plentiful:

- Infant mortality rate increases in infants born to mothers with less education.
- Cancer mortality is higher among African Americans than whites.
- Tooth decay with resultant decreased quality of life is nearly twice as likely in children living below the poverty level.
- Injuries and suicide are more common in American Indian and Alaskan Native males.
- Lower socioeconomic status increases the risk of diabetes, cardiovascular disease, chronic respiratory disease, cervical cancer, and mental distress.

While the root causes of these divisions are numerous—including poverty, food insecurity, housing insecurity, lack of insurance, racism, classism, and other structural inequities—one root cause that isn't discussed enough is health literacy.

I've seen over and over again that individuals with the same resources—same amount of money, same level of education, same race and ethnicity—can experience very different outcomes based on how familiar they are with navigating health-care systems. This knowledge gained from prior experience can be invaluable, but it shouldn't have to be this way.

Ed is the parent of two children. His eldest was in the NICU for difficulty breathing and feeding due to congenital heart disease. Ed made it through several hospitalizations, emergency room visits, specialist visits, and physical therapy. In the process, he got to know the pediatrician, who introduced him to a social worker at the hospital. His social worker helped him learn about prior authorizations, co-pays, insurance advocates, and about legal protections for parents in the workplace and children's rights to appropriate education.

Ed's second child has a peanut allergy. After his first reaction and the subsequent ER visit, Ed sought out expert advice on how best to manage the peanut allergy from the right doctors and found peer-parent support. The family has had to learn to read all the ingredient labels and be vigilant against accidental exposure. Ed had to spend a few hours fighting with insurance to get enough epinephrine injectors so one could be left at school in the event of an emergency, and the pediatrician had to fill out a lot of forms, but he knew that process from all the forms and insurance paperwork they navigated with their first child. His second child's peanut allergy has been a lot for the family to deal with, but overall, they have taken it in stride largely because they found the help they needed along the way.

Carmela, a first-time parent, took her child to the ER for what she thought to be a rash. When he was diagnosed with a food allergy, it didn't really make sense to Carmela. She thought food allergies were serious, with trouble breathing and a swollen mouth. The rash seemed more like a nuisance, on the level of a bugbite. The ER doctor and Carmela also could not determine exactly which food might have been involved, though they narrowed it to two. Since he had eaten both of those foods in the past without a problem, a serious food allergy seemed even less likely to Carmela.

By the time they were seen in the ER, it was late, and Carmela was exhausted. She didn't really know what to ask about, what this diagnosis and medication meant. She didn't have faith that the ER doctor really knew what he was talking about, since he didn't seem to listen to her and even called her child the wrong name when going through the discharge paperwork. Her mother was lactose intolerant, and she assumed this food allergy was similar. She decided to simply minimize the exposure to the same foods the child had that day. She was not given any cream to help her child's rash, but was prescribed another medication, an epinephrine auto-injector used for anaphylaxis, which wasn't automatically covered by insurance and was really expensive. She hesitated to fill the medication, and when in the days following the ER visit, she saw her child improve without the medication, she figured she wouldn't need to fill the medication after all.

In the weeks that followed, Carmela was scared the rash would recur and limited his exposure to a handful of foods that she knew were not related to the prior rash. She read about elimination diets online and thought it made sense to reintroduce one food at a time to ensure those didn't worsen the rash. But because Carmela's plan was a little complicated and she wasn't sure what to tell her babysitter, the babysitter didn't really know what was going on. Then the babysitter gave Carmela's child candy containing peanuts. This time he ended up back in the ER with a rash, swelling around his mouth, and difficulty breathing. Now Carmela understands that her child has a definite diagnosis of a food allergy. She was fully counseled and received instructions and a clear plan, but she also feels scared to feed her child anything or leave him with childcare or at school. She still isn't sure how to afford the medication.

So, is Carmela a bad parent? Did she do something wrong? These aren't the right questions to ask. Often, our inclination is to put all the pressure on the parent, without accounting for the fact that every family brings their own resources to the situation. In our examples, Ed started out with valuable knowledge and experience, undoubtedly learned the hard way, that helped him know how to communicate with his child's doctors, how to seek out resources for his child, and implement a plan that worked. It's not Carmela's fault that her child landed back in the ER. She did not have the knowledge and support she needed.

There is no standardized curriculum, in our public education system or elsewhere, that offers people valuable information about how to navigate medical and educational institutions. Parents come to their care professionals with varying amounts of resources and knowledge. And the health-care system is not universally set up to teach health literacy to all. This may leave many parents feeling lost at sea, but this is a gap that I can begin to address in this book.

I can't tell you how many times friends have called me after leaving an appointment questioning the plan they were given. They will ask, "Do you really think medication is necessary?" or, "Kelly, my doctor says I need to see a specialist. Is this a big deal? Should I be worried?" In other circumstances, my friends will be very worried about an issue and jump right to a specialist without speaking with their primary care doctor. Sometimes this helps expedite access, but more often it winds up delaying or confusing care. Issues like asthma and constipation, for example, require a fair amount of monitoring and bidirectional communication best suited for a primary care doctor, though of course there are situations where pulmonologists and gastroenterologists can help confirm the diagnosis or optimize the plan.

It's not in my ability to change the health-care system, particularly in the United States, where more resources are desperately needed to support families with challenges. What I can do is help families better advocate for themselves by providing a primer on where families often get stuck. As part of efforts to promote efficiency and improve quality of care, there are a lot of protocols for how the medical system deals with medical diagnoses. I understand that sometimes, it's almost as if the doctor's office is a black box. Insert your symptoms and physical exam findings, and the medical industrial complex will spit out your plan.

This system might work well for typical people facing typical problems. If you have fever and a sore throat and need a strep-throat test and antibiotics, the protocol will just spit out the right plan for you. However, at its core, managing challenges and working with people is as much an art as a science. If no one talks to you, no one will uncover the fact that this is your fourth time having strep throat in a year and that you snore loudly. Maybe your tonsils need to come out. Or maybe your diet is very restricted, and your immune system isn't functioning properly. The moment things stray off the protocol, even in minor ways, you begin to face closed doors and mixed messages. The reason this adherence to cookie-cutter care is so baffling is that most people don't fit the typical mold—as an example, nearly 40 percent of school-age children have a chronic condition.

I have a vague memory of one of my last visits to my own pediatrician, before I went off to college. They explained to me how I should approach my medical care as an adult—essentially that I should always tell the provider my full medical history—even if I didn't know how it might be relevant. While I think of this as good advice, my own history never really fits on the form in the right boxes, and many times a nurse abbreviates my history for quick review by the doctor. There is an important context to your child's care, and the medical team only sees a fraction of it. Families take these plans, the medications, referrals, and whatever else and incorporate it into the rest of their lives. There's a bigger picture for these patients, including their identities and values and hobbies. This is why you need a road map so you can advocate for your child and yourself.

If you've been dealing with your specific challenge for a while, it's likely you have encountered some of this stuff—your doctor has given you prescriptions and referrals or your educational assessment team has given you an individualized education plan. I would love to contextualize what these pieces of the plan can *really* mean for the people involved. By reviewing this general information and seeing my perspective, you might learn something to help your child and your family.

The Medical System

Many pediatricians schedule four patients an hour: two well-child visits and two focused sick visits. These are typically scheduled with the well-child visits allotted twenty-five minutes and the sick visits allotted ten minutes. If you do the math, you'll note that this makes for seventy minutes in a sixty-minute hour, but some of the work is done by the assistants or nurses taking vital signs, performing hearing and vision tests, or giving vaccinations, so mostly it works out.

Within the visits, a lot needs to happen. At a well-child visit, the doctor does a full physical exam and assesses nutrition, growth, lead exposure, development, behavior, mental health, sleep, skin care, body image, and a number of other things. Just one of these topics could fill twenty-five minutes, but inevitably more comes up, too. Insurance covers a well-child visit intended to address typical preventive health-care needs for no additional cost. This means that routine screenings are included, but should a diagnosis arise from these screenings like a developmental delay, hearing loss, or depression, the care of these conditions is not included and generates a separate bill. Most families would prefer to discuss common and ongoing problems like seasonal allergies and eczema within the "free" annual visit, but this is not the way the system is designed. Technically, if a pediatrician addresses other concerns in addition to a preventive visit, they are required to include additional billing codes. Ideally, addressing these additional concerns would also allocate additional time on the schedule—to discuss the situation, educate the family, and recommend any additional workup or referrals.

Publicly accessible insurance policies like managed-care Medicaid reimburse the annual preventive visit for about ninety dollars in most states. Private insurance reimbursement is typically more and not public knowledge. Half of that typically goes to overhead—fixed costs of facilities and staff. So, the doctor makes about forty-five dollars to manage your child's case year-round. To earn their salary as the lowest paid physicians, most pediatricians must see a lot of patients. This means a full-time pediatrician on average manages a panel of over 1,500 children a year.[2]

Pediatricians also have lots of work that needs to be done outside of the traditional visit: telephone calls, emails, school and camp forms, prescription refills, prior authorizations, care coordination, and more. Doctors try to squeeze this work in when there are no-show visits or on nights and weekends. In some cases, these tasks are delegated to nurses, medical assistants, and other members of the care team. But since this work is generally unpaid, it's typically not seen as a priority. Still, for most pediatricians, these tasks take about a quarter of their time. All families see the value in this unpaid work; you need this stuff done to help your children, and pediatricians know this and try to help.

I once treated a sweet little boy named Mike, who had been born after just twenty-eight weeks of pregnancy. He had done very well after NICU discharge but had an undescended testicle for which he needed surgery. He had also struggled with frequent ear infections and needed ear tubes inserted to prevent further infections. His parents were rightfully concerned about these two procedures. As a preterm infant, anesthesia might irritate his lungs. They knew the procedures were medically necessary, but couldn't they be combined? Both surgeons agreed in theory, but someone needed to work out the details. Every third Thursday, both surgeons operated at the children's hospital; otherwise, their schedules didn't overlap. But the surgeons used different operating rooms and different staff, so someone had to get both teams to talk to each other. Could I help?

Of course, as Mike's pediatrician, I knew it was best practice to minimize exposures to anesthesia. I would help, but it took about ten phone calls and ten hours of my time. Then Mike got sick right before the procedure—just a cold, but we still had to postpone. Rescheduling took another forty-five minutes. For Mike and his family, this work had value. If we couldn't consolidate the procedures, Mike would face two doses of anesthesia instead of one. Eventually, the insurance company agreed to combine the procedures into one day. But the unpaid work to make it happen was done entirely on lunch breaks and borrowed time. Had there been a few poorly timed emergencies, or had I been out of the office on vacation, Mike might have ended up having two procedures.

So, pediatricians are human and have finite hours in the day to help their patients. At the same time, it's understandable that most families end up frustrated after visits. There's not enough time, not enough attention, and not enough follow-up devoted to important issues relevant to a family's life. I do have hope that with time, reimbursement models for health insurance should adjust to pay for this type of work. In recent years, new billing codes have been established for care coordination and telemedicine visits, though reimbursement remains murky.

In the meantime, you should be aware that every office and every doctor handles this work differently. In my complex-care practice, my hospital employed Rose, a patient care coordinator; Jillian, a registered nurse; and Allison, a licensed social worker. In our practice, if you had an issue with transportation or getting an appointment, you needed Rose. For an insurance authorization issue or need for skilled nursing services at home, you needed Allison. For medication difficulty or a technology issue, you needed Jillian. We worked as a team, and while generally speaking, the staff and the families benefited from the expertise of a larger team, there was a learning curve and a bit of confusion for families as they learned who could help with what. Later, when I joined a small private practice, we had a smaller team—just my patient care coordinator Liz and me. Depending on the family's needs, one model might be better than the other, more direct attention from a physician or more support from social workers and nurses who can advance your care in other important ways.

For routine well visits, any office can typically handle your needs. But when your child is facing a challenge, it's helpful to know who does what within the office. If you have a problem with a referral or need a form or a prescription, who do you contact? The more you can anticipate these needs, the more efficiently and effectively you can get the help you need. Consider the following as you collaborate with your pediatrician:

- When you have a complex follow-up question, be sure to schedule an appointment. While a co-pay is an inconvenience, the quality of the advice you receive will likely be more robust when you have the undivided time and attention of your doctor.
- If you aren't sure if your pediatrician has sufficient experience with your child's condition, ask. Like any professional, pediatricians have strengths and weaknesses, and if your condition is outside their scope, they may recommend resources to bridge any gaps, such as working closely with a specialist or early-intervention provider.
- Understand how the office works before a need arises. How do referrals go through? What's the process or the turnaround time for a school form or medication refill? Who answers the phones after hours for an emergency? Does the pediatrician share records with specialists and receive reports back from them routinely?

I know many people feel a deep allegiance to their pediatrician, and I hope your pediatrician can be a key support. However, in many circumstances, the factors that were most important in choosing a pediatrician before the diagnosis change after the diagnosis is determined. Perhaps convenience and a low co-pay were how you ended up with a practice, but now you want or need someone with more expertise in your area or who is more accessible. Some pediatricians and their offices tend to adapt to the unique needs of some families better than others. Consider if the person you chose originally remains the right person.

Pediatricians care for their patients, and sometimes we are sad when families leave, but, if you think it's best for your family, please don't hesitate to move on. You can also provide some feedback to your pediatrician such as, "I love this practice, but I can't come for an in-person visit every time I need a new referral or have a question pop up (which feels like always). I will have to find a practice that offers remote ways I can communicate with the care team." This may solve your problem by motivating change, or your doctor may admit the practice isn't well-suited to your needs, in which case maybe they know an alternative practice that will be a better fit for you.

Prioritizing your needs doesn't end with picking a pediatrician. Another common part of the plan is medication. In my experience, medication sounds simple and expected, but often is more difficult than families anticipate.

Medication

Not long ago, a friend and I were discussing his son's challenges with focus and learning. I had initially raised the possibility of inattentive attention deficit hyperactivity disorder (ADHD). Most people might consider ADHD children as those who are "bouncing off the walls," but children with inattentive ADHD often elude diagnosis because an observer can't always know if the child is distracted on the inside. My friend hadn't really considered it, but after doing some research he saw that the diagnosis might fit his son. In the weeks following, he had a dozen conversations with babysitters, friends, and teachers about his son's strengths and struggles.

His gym teacher had noticed his son was often missing directions and needed them repeated. Parents of his friends had noticed that while most kids on a playdate could stick with one activity for a longer period, he frequently seemed to wander, engaging more superficially in play. His teachers thought he was "keeping up, but capable of more." The observations enriched my friend's understanding and validated his concerns. He saw his day-to-day behavior through a different lens. He made an appointment with a doctor, and subsequently a psychiatrist who provided more information, evaluated his son, and eventually agreed with the diagnosis and prescribed a stimulant medication.

When he arrived home with the firm diagnosis and the medication, his husband was extremely uncertain. For his husband, accepting a medication meant accepting a complex and chronic diagnosis. Most everyone acknowledges that medication is sometimes necessary to help a sick child, but most parents dislike the idea of giving their child medication. In practice, daily medication administration is a struggle—kids don't want to take it, remembering to give it takes energy, and keeping the medication stocked and stored safely is more work. We worry about side effects and other risks. But medication is sometimes necessary. More than that, medication can be lifesaving. For this little boy, it would enrich his ability to learn, play, and make friends.

He called me about his partner's hesitations and asked, "Can't you talk to him and explain this?" I happily agreed to do so; he is my friend too. But I encouraged my friend to see that he had been gathering the information and opinions and resources for months to get to a place where he saw the necessity and utility of medication. So, while he had kept his husband abreast of the news, he hadn't been as invested in the process or heard from any of those professionals directly about their perspectives. I spoke to the hesitant partner briefly and encouraged him to dig in with some of the care team, the teachers, therapists, and doctors who had evaluated his son, so he could hear firsthand how this had come about. After a few conversations and a couple of weeks to digest the new information, both parents were on board with the trial of medication. The next time I saw the family a few months later, both parents shared enthusiastically that their son was thriving; medication had helped him to engage in school and friendships in a more robust way. While there was still work to do, accepting the diagnosis and need for medication had been an essential step for his well-being.

Often it takes time, research, and education to accept a diagnosis and accept the necessity and safety of medication. Even if you are on board with medication, often your co-parent, babysitters, or the child's grandparents haven't had an opportunity to receive education or counseling or ask any questions. It's asking a lot for one parent to assume the responsibility to educate and inform other stakeholders in your family about medication. If this is your situation, I encourage you not to hesitate to ask your pediatrician for resources to share with the rest of your circle.

Central to understanding medication is also understanding the goals of treatment. Will my child be on this medication forever? Will this fix the problem? What are the side effects, and will the benefit of the medication really be worth the side effects? Additionally, what if the medication doesn't seem to work, what will the alternatives be? Beginning a medication often feels like a big commitment.

When we consider medication, there are a few best practices you should know. Most medication is temperature sensitive, so storing it in your car, bathroom, or kitchen may degrade it over time. Some medications are light sensitive and shouldn't be exposed to sun. Some liquid medications, especially those reconstituted from powder by a pharmacist like antibiotics, often need to be shaken before the dose is pulled out. Calculating the correct dose is very important, and using milliliters instead of "spoons" is always a safer way to measure.

Taking medication daily long-term without missing a dose is very challenging, and on average, adults only take it correctly half the time.[3] Giving medication to children who have tantrums and preferences about taste and texture can be even more difficult. Even studies about medication adherence consider taking your medication 80 percent of the time to be good (though I'd encourage you to aim higher, as we know taking medication is required for it to work!). Failure to improve on medication sometimes leads to physicians using medications with more side effects or risk. We know that adhering to a regimen of medication is difficult for most people, and nonadherence at the population level is an enormous public health challenge.[4] If you haven't been able to give the medication to your child regularly, when you see your doctor for follow-up, be honest.

Once you are ready to begin, there are a few practical ways to make giving medication easier:

- Ensure that the schedule assigned by the doctor will work for your family. If something worries you, speak up. Avoid medications that need to be taken four times a day if at all possible. If the dosing schedule seems too frequent to be practical for your family, discuss alternatives with your child's doctors.

- Ask for advice on administering the medication from a doctor, nurse, or pharmacist who knows the specifics of your child's age, flavor and texture preferences, and the available medication options. Some children vigorously protest liquid medication and may do better with a tablet that can be crushed or a capsule that can be opened and given on a spoon of food.
- Learning how best to administer medication is important, especially for nasal sprays, eye drops, inhalers, and prescription creams. For conditions requiring emergency treatment like asthma, epilepsy, and food allergies, it's essential that all caregivers have an opportunity to practice.
- Strategies to help you remember to take each dose include the following: Tie medicine time to a solid part of your routine (for example, before breakfast or when you brush your teeth). Use technology like phone alarms. Consider physical reminders like daily pill packs and stickers (one company called tooktake has cute ones where you remove a tab for every dose you take!). I have had kids keep their preventive asthma inhalers in their shoes for school so they have to take it out to put them on in the morning (and hopefully remember to then take their daily medication dose before leaving the house).

If your child is mature enough to begin assuming the responsibility for taking medication, great. But consider that supervision will likely be necessary for a long time, probably for years. I compare this to potty training. While your child may have been toilet trained by age three, you probably still encouraged them to go to the bathroom before big outings for much longer. If the medication is truly important, it requires adult supervision.

Referrals

Imagine that your baby has bad reflux and is very fussy. In a sleep-deprived haze you look to your pediatrician for guidance and are handed a slip of paper with a name and number. What does this mean?

Some parents interpret referrals as a brush-off. You might think, "My primary care doctor is sick of me." Or maybe you'll think, "My doctor must be stumped and has no idea," or, "This must be really serious if we need to see a specialist." I have found that even very savvy parents did not understand why they were being sent elsewhere.

All primary care physicians use referrals. It's frequently said that primary care physicians know a little about a lot. I like to think we know a lot about a lot, but one of the most important things is that we know when we need help from other specialists.

Your pediatrician makes referrals for good reasons, and everyone on the team should know what they are. Some referrals are done to facilitate a diagnosis. Maybe your pediatrician suspects your fussy baby as having a milk-protein allergy but wants the gastroenterologist to weigh in and confirm the diagnosis before restricting the diet. If your child is older with significant reflux, the referral may be for endoscopy—a procedure to evaluate the anatomy and rule out a condition known as eosinophilic esophagitis. If your primary care doctor is concerned about this, the only way to firmly make the diagnosis is by a procedure done by a gastroenterologist. The specialist needs to look at the lining of the esophagus. These referrals are often intended as one-off consultations.

Other referrals are made for long-term management. If your child has inflammatory bowel disease, a congenital heart defect, or a combined diagnosis of ADHD and learning disabilities, the relevant specialist may own the care of the condition. This means the specialist will do an initial evaluation and send notes to your pediatrician for their reference, but the specialist will be in charge of the follow-up plan.

Whatever the reason, you need to know why you are being referred so you know what to expect. Who is going to help you? How will communication work? What will your appointment schedule look like? While it may initially feel dismissive to receive instructions that your issue is now some other doctor's issue, I encourage you to see referrals as respectful. Your doctor thinks your problem requires additional resources and wants to help you get those resources. Understanding why you are being referred will also allow you to express your opinion. Perhaps you prefer that the gastroenterologist manage your child's reflux long-term and the attention of a specialist and added visits feel helpful to your family. Or maybe you would prefer your pediatrician manage the reflux and send you back to the specialist only if reevaluation of the medical issue is necessary due to your child's specific symptoms. Understanding the way referrals work can allow you to express your preferences.

When your child is referred, I encourage you to ask a lot of questions. Some are very important. In particular:

- How soon should the appointment happen?
- Is this specific person ideal, or would any physician in this specialty suffice?
- What will happen going forward?
- If you have an emergency, who should you call? The pediatrician, the specialist, urgent care, or the ER?
- How will the specialist and the doctor communicate?
- Who will renew the medication and handle relevant school forms?

Understanding how the specialist fits into your care will also help you ensure you pick the right one. For a one-off evaluation to access testing—for example, a child with a murmur that sounds benign but warrants further investigation with an echocardiogram—it may matter less who the specialist is. In this situation, you should prioritize convenience and ease of communication with the primary doctor. For a one-off diagnostic evaluation—for example, a child with concern for intoeing who is recommended to see an orthopedist—especially when the urgency is low, it's worth waiting for or traveling to see the best-qualified individual. Since it's likely to be only one visit, the location of the specialist will not matter so much.

When you are referred for long-term management or a specialized procedure, the choice of specialist becomes a more important decision. Ask your doctor and the specialist:

- How does the specialist's expertise relate to your issue?
- What volume of this type of problem does the specialist see?
- Is this the type of problem that will require frequent visits, where you should consider travel convenience?

Specialty Centers

Studies show that in many areas of specialty surgery, outcomes for patients are better in high-volume centers. When the surgeon and hospital teams have more experience, it's no surprise that there will be better outcomes and fewer errors.[5] This matters most for the most complex surgeries, such as surgeries to correct higher complexity congenital heart defects. In these situations, you should strongly consider the most qualified specialist, even if the location is somewhat inconvenient.

Subspecialized multidisciplinary clinics are increasingly popping up to meet the needs of children with complex medical conditions. For example, a clinic designed for children with cerebral palsy may include a general pediatrician, an orthopedist, a neurologist, and a pediatric rehabilitation specialist. These physicians would work collaboratively to help a family decide a plan. When there is a good match between a child's needs and the design of the clinic, these clinics can combine several referrals into one place, providing a "one-stop shop." Though it can make for a long, tiring day, it's much easier to take off a day of work if you can have four appointments done in one day than to try and arrange four separate days off work. Additionally, having all the relevant specialists in one room can enrich the conversation, enabling families to access a better quality of care. Without a combined clinic, a family might see the pediatric rehabilitation specialist who recommends braces and then later see an orthopedist who recommends surgery and feel lost and confused. When the specialists work in a team setting, they can negotiate a plan together with a family's input, agreeing to, say, a plan of trying bracing for six months and anticipating surgery in a year if no improvement. When care is centralized this way, it may be easier for the care team to communicate and keep track of records and your child's medical history. Additionally, these clinics are often housed within academic centers, and the specialists who have a vested interest in just your challenge can find it easier to keep up-to-date with the latest research.

Centers of excellence are common for conditions like cystic fibrosis, diabetes, inflammatory bowel disease, and children with a history of extremely preterm birth. These conditions often require coordinated access to multiple specialists like pulmonology, nutrition, gastroenterology, endocrinology, and development. Additionally, many genetic conditions have centers where children with trisomy 21, Williams syndrome, Turner's syndrome, Prader-Willi, or others may be seen exclusively. In their local community, many of these children may be the only child with this diagnosis their pediatrician or school has seen, but these centers gather hundreds of children and learn from their experiences in a way that can promote the quality of medical care and create a sense of community.

As a survivor of pediatric cancer, I continued to travel to North Carolina to see my pediatric oncologist for regular follow-ups until my midthirties. After having chemotherapy and radiation at a young age, I need routine testing to monitor for complications due to the toxicities of the therapies I received. I also need surveillance for secondary malignancies. As a young adult, I could have tried to manage moving this care to Cambridge, Massachusetts, when in college, Spain when I studied abroad, or New York after I graduated. But the specialized survivorship program in my home state of North Carolina had advantages, including plans and protocols in place to ensure all the follow-ups happened. They had all my records and imaging for reference, and I knew if I tried to transition to a regular doctor, all the work of keeping that organized would fall on me.

For many families, it's worth considering whether the cost, stress, and inconvenience of traveling for care is worth the benefit. If you can find the right fit of a specialized clinic, it may make your life easier and improve the quality of care, even if it's distant from your home. To find a clinic that fits your family's needs, you can ask your doctor, investigate what the bigger children's hospitals in your area offer, learn from non-profits devoted to research and advocacy for your child's condition, or seek support from a family-to-family health information center locally through Family Voices. This type of research may be intimidating, but I'll go into more detail about how to make it more manageable later in Chapter 13.

Multiple Cooks in the Kitchen

Eating and growing is the primary metabolic demand for a little baby. So, when their heart function is low, as it is for babies with congenital heart disease, they often have difficulty eating due to fatigue. When they can't eat well, they get insufficient calories to grow bigger and stronger. These children end up seeing a gastroenterologist to help maximize calories and optimize feeding. Then the cardiologists and cardiac surgeons think about the best time to do corrective surgery and how to adjust medications to improve heart function. But frequently, the parents end up confused. The gastroenterologist tells them, "We can't improve your child's feeding until your child gets the heart intervention needed to get strong enough to eat more." Then the cardiologist says, "Go back to the gastroenterologist; we can't do a heart intervention until your child reaches a certain size." And the parents would cry and come to see me feeling hopeless.

Because my complex-care practice had more time with families and more nursing and social work support, I could fully explore the details of the situation to help ensure that these babies were really getting the maximum nutrition support possible. Often I would advocate for the family by getting the gastroenterologist and the cardiologist to speak with each other directly. Without a medical quarterback, these families would ping-pong between the gastroenterologist and the cardiologist. When I could support improved communication, all the specialists could come together with the family and come up with a plan to meet everyone's needs. Often this required buy-in from everyone; my team would help the family get more hours of skilled nursing support to facilitate the feeds at home, gastroenterology would come up with a creative way to get more nutrition into the child, and cardiology would either recommend a medication to promote the child's stamina or reduce the weight requirement for surgery to something more within reach.

When many doctors are involved in managing an issue, inevitably there will be disagreements. Each physician approaches the child's situation with his or her own perspective grounded in their medical expertise, their values, and their personalities. Sometimes medicine is more of an art than a science, and two physicians may make two different plans for the same child based on the same data. While it can feel black and white— one doctor must be right and the other must be wrong—truthfully, the answer is more in the gray.

When the stakeholders in your child's care seem to disagree about the best way to move forward, encouraging an open discussion of the issues at hand is best. Often, there is a simple explanation; a doctor may admit that the other plan is equally appropriate or even better than the one he suggested. Other times, you may learn that one doctor had a piece of data the other didn't, and that piece of information, whether it was a facet of the history or a lab or imaging result, led him to make the decision for a good reason. Most physicians went into medicine to help people, and when you push back on the plan they suggest with a constructive intent—to clarify their thinking or understand why someone disagrees—often you may find they are willing to help. Sometimes you'll see that the gray zone allows you as a parent to make the decision based on your values and priorities.

The same issue applies when educators or mental health professionals are collaborating in your child's care. If doctor-to-doctor communication can be difficult, communication with teachers and therapists can be even more challenging. These professionals sometimes have no time blocked from their weekly schedule for administrative tasks like communicating with an outside doctor. They often do not share a language for how they think about the child's condition.

Imagine Marnie, the single parent to a vivacious and rambunctious young boy, Nate, who carries a diagnosis of attention deficit hyperactivity disorder. Prior to making the diagnosis, Nate had an intensive evaluation with a child-development specialist who helped exclude the possibility of comorbid learning disabilities or other mental health issues like anxiety. For Nate's ongoing care, Marnie gets feedback from his teachers, who primarily want him to learn and participate productively in the classroom setting. Nate is also working with an occupational therapist outside of the school system who is supporting his executive function skills to optimize his day-to-day functioning—organizing his homework and getting himself out the door in the morning. Marnie gets feedback from these two on a weekly basis, and then every two to three months she sees the pediatrician who is primarily charged with renewing or adjusting Nate's medication. This plan seems to be going well, until all of a sudden, it's not.

Nate is thriving at home and his work with the private occupational therapist has him accomplishing tasks he previously struggled with, but at school the teacher is seeing something different. After lunch, Nate loses focus and acts out, distracting the class. The teacher tried a few ways to improve his behavior, but the principal had to get involved when an episode escalated. The teacher feels overall that Marnie should consider more medication or a different dose to support him more appropriately in the afternoon. Now Marnie, in addition to reacting to this news as any parent might—maybe feeling disappointed, defensive, or upset—also has to serve as Nate's quarterback, communicating what's happening at school with the occupational therapist and doctor involved.

To support Marnie in this work, I recommend the following:

- Keep notes. It's helpful to keep a journal of the feedback. Just a date with a brief summary of their remarks will likely be adequate, but when things are going in the wrong direction, make your notes more detailed with direct quotes.

- Ask questions to learn as much information as you can. Especially if you aren't at school, you may not know if the curriculum has shifted in a way that your child is struggling with or if there is a social situation with peers complicating things. Even simple considerations like how his eating is at lunch may be relevant.

- When people involved with your child disagree, encourage them to speak directly. If the occupational therapist insists that Nate is doing well on his current medication, maybe they can ask the teacher what techniques are used at school to help his behavior and make some specific recommendations.

- Be open to the fact that everyone's observations have value. A child may behave differently in different circumstances and it's likely you can learn from the teacher's observations.

We are often quick to add additional resources to a situation where a child is struggling. More perspectives and more insights are additive. But managing a bigger team is more work. Sometimes you can outsource this care-coordination work to a member of your team—your pediatrician, a social worker, a member of an IEP team, a nurse who works for your insurance company. This delegation can work especially well when there is a disagreement you can point your finger at—this doctor recommends this procedure and this one doesn't: What should we do?

But often this care-coordination work falls on you as a parent. Identifying that this skilled work has value for your child and your family is an important step. It takes time and energy. This book will help you learn your options, your rights, and strategies to do necessary research, stay organized, and communicate your needs.

Follow-Up Visits

James was a five-year-old boy who was doing really well. He had congenital heart disease and had been through a few surgeries, though now his heart was "fixed." Before his heart had been repaired, he had had several hospitalizations for respiratory infections. We had tried treating asthma and allergies, though it hadn't made much difference. He once had a lung infection that required a surgical procedure to drain a collection of infected fluid pockets in his chest.

Because of the severity of his illnesses, he had seen a pulmonologist, an allergist, and an infectious disease specialist. James had been slow to achieve developmental milestones amid the surgeries and illnesses, so he also saw a developmental specialist. He had been slow to gain weight and at one point required a feeding tube, so he still saw a gastroenterologist, though his growth recently had been excellent. He also needed glasses, like everyone else in his family.

All this aside, James was mostly doing better after his heart surgery. He hadn't had a significant respiratory infection in a year, nor did he have many remaining signs of asthma or allergies. His weight gain and growth had been excellent since his last cardiac surgery, and his last few cardiology notes were quite optimistic. He had missed a few appointments with me and had not yet gotten vaccinations typically given at five years of age. Then his school refused to let him come back, due to a mandate for the vaccines—and James's family had not filed for an exemption.

So, I saw James for an urgent well-child visit so he could go back to school and so that the parents could get back to work. I was looking forward to seeing him, as I thought he had been doing so well. When I walked in, the dad looked very upset. I had a nurse play with James while I took the father to my office to discuss matters.

This "urgent" nonurgent visit had been the last straw at work and his supervisor had threatened to let him go. James's family had accrued a lot of debt when their son was in and out of the hospital, and now that things were more stable, Mom and Dad were both burning the candle at both ends and working multiple jobs to try to catch up financially. Even though James had progressed, he still had a lot of appointments—with the eye doctor, dentist, gastroenterologist, nutritionist, asthma specialist, allergy specialist, and cardiologist. Each appointment required a parent to take time off work and for James to miss school, and he was already behind academically. And none of these appointments had accomplished what the family needed most, which was to clear James for school. The family needed him to go to school, for his educational and developmental benefit, and to provide consistent childcare.

As James's primary care doctor, I felt terrible. While I had entered the visit proud about James's improvement, thinking I had helped him get to a more stable, better place, this family didn't have the support they needed. I had gotten them 90 percent of the way there, and then dropped the ball. How was the family supposed to know which follow-ups were necessary and which were not without my help?

When working with physicians, there are standard office workflows. Once you're seen for a consultation, you return every few months to check in. These follow-up visits add value to your care by making sure things are improving or stable and allowing for a reassessment to adjust treatment plans to fit a child's care. But specialists aren't mind readers. In James's case, they did not know his respiratory status had improved so significantly, and the visits could be spaced out or deferred until he had an issue.

Specialists often don't have the long-term relationship or big picture to know the context of the visit within the family's life. Practically speaking, most specialists are concerned with optimizing patient outcomes. Imagine a child with asthma on a maintenance inhaler. The pulmonologist can't reliably predict if, as the seasons change and the child grows, the asthma might get better or worse. The pulmonologist may have an idea of what new drugs are going to come on the market or what guidelines from professional societies might change, and so coming back for another visit gives an opportunity for reevaluation and a chance to consider if the child's status or the scientific consensus changed. A specialist may say that if one hundred follow-up visits result in finding one child who needs a major change in the plan and twenty who need a minor tweak, it's reasonable. Specialists don't get any incentive to say, "Don't come back"; instead, they only take on risk.

From James's family's perspective, having a 1 percent chance of substantially changing the plan based on the visit might feel like a big waste of time. If the specialists knew the larger context of the parents' work constraints, they might have adjusted the expectations for follow-ups and encouraged them to decide when it was necessary. I knew that James's family had other commitments, which is why I had spaced out my own visits with him. We had a relationship, and I knew they would call me if they needed help between routine visits. But I didn't know how burdensome the specialist follow-ups had been on the family, and had I known this earlier, I would have helped the family determine which of the six subspecialty appointments were high priority and which could be skipped. Or I might have been able to identify resources like intermittent family medical leave, which would have provided a layer of protection for James's father. That day, I offered to write a letter or call James's father's supervisor to explain the situation as well as the fact that I anticipated that there would be fewer schedule interruptions going forward, but James's father refused. Like many, he valued his privacy and didn't want to make excuses about his work. Luckily, the threat was just a threat, and his employer did not follow through with letting him go. The family was able to get to a financially more secure place, with James well enough to allow both parents to work. But I learned a lesson that day, and I began to make it a habit to ask parents how their child's illness was impacting their career earlier and more often, as well as request social work assistance to support families in maximizing their job protections.

Doctors will always offer lots of attention when things aren't going well or in times of crisis. We choose this profession to help those in need. But when things are going well, our attention moves on to other children who need our help. Where does this leave the children who are doing well? Their needs should still receive care and attention. This dilemma underscores the need for parents to become their own family's advocates.

Having been a patient myself, I've sat in my paper gown uncomfortably perched on exam tables while a doctor dressed in slacks, a tie, and a white coat stood above me. As much as things are moving away from this power dynamic of a doctor dictating a patient's care, I know that there is still pressure on patients to go along with what they are told. Doctors tell parents to do X, Y, and Z, and often parents just do those things without questioning or pushing back at every step. Increasingly, parents are encouraged to find the best doctor for their family and research their treatment options, but follow-up appointments are another topic we should question.

We all agree that children's play time, nap time, and school time are all important. Parents need time to attend to these needs. And time for paid and unpaid work is also valuable. And we do not want to waste any time. As James's story illustrates, parent advocacy about the family's time would have allowed me to advise on how to decrease the number of specialist visits and reduce the strain on the family overall.

I encourage you to ask a lot of questions about the visits you are planning so you can see how they fit or don't fit into your goals of care and your big picture:

- What's the goal of this appointment?
- What are the alternatives? Could I email you updated weights or blood pressures to allow us to push the next visit out further?
- What's the risk or cost of putting it off?
- Could my primary care doctor take over the responsibility of monitoring my child's progress?
- Can I cancel the routine follow-up appointment if there are no further issues? Could we switch to coming in only when issues arise?

Remember, we're all working toward the same goal of supporting your family, and you as the parent are the best one to decide how that looks.

Navigating Mental Health Services

I had a telemedicine consultation with a patient—Sarah, a nine-year-old girl—who had "something going on." Her mother described how Sarah would ruminate on her fears of new experiences, sometimes even months before the event of concern. Would she make friends at art camp? Would she be the worst artist there? Would she be alone at lunch time? Would they use materials she was unfamiliar with? The week before camp, she would have trouble sleeping and she would melt down over minor issues. If dinner wasn't her favorite, she'd get explosively angry and throw things. These behaviors all seemed out of character for her. School conferences had recently taken place, and the teacher had shared her concerns too. Sarah was increasingly withdrawing from her peers and hesitant to engage in activities she hadn't yet mastered.

The consultation was not meant to help the family understand the diagnosis—the parents had already come to the conclusion that Sarah had excessive anxiety. Sarah's mom had faced her own anxiety and struggled for years to find the right support for herself. What Mom asked for now, through tears, was how to find the right help for her daughter, fast. While this is such a common story, getting that help still isn't an easy task.

Finding high-quality, evidence-based, affordable, and racially and culturally sensitive behavioral health care can be a challenge. In 2016, an estimated one out of five American children had a mental health diagnosis and half did not receive any treatment.[6] The reason for these gaps and barriers to care are numerous. We have a shortage of providers—too few individuals trained to provide needed evaluation and treatment in many communities. Our insurance system provides inadequate reimbursement, leading many practices to offer services for additional out-of-pocket fees or not take insurance at all. These expenses are often out of reach for most families. We have limited and inconsistent availability of treatments for children of all abilities and ages and of evidence-based treatments like parent–child interaction therapy and cognitive behavioral therapy. For families, the decision to pursue behavioral health support requires them to accept the need for services and reconcile the persistent (if decreasing) stigma against those with mental health challenges. There are real logistic hurdles to jump—finding a practice, navigating the wait list, and making the time commitment of therapy are all significant burdens. Weekly appointments require a lot of parent support, including transportation, often on workdays, particularly when school-based services aren't an option.

One of the most important things you can do is seek help early. Because of shortages in qualified providers and mismatches between rural demand and urban supply, wait lists can be months long. Centers associated with academic institutions can provide an excellent quality of care once you are within the system, but it's not uncommon that the intake process takes months. Not every office is suited for every condition, and many offices do not take insurance.

A primary consideration is cost. When we consider the cost of a medication, it's often straightforward and covered by insurance. But when we speak of therapy, the cost of the service, while often significant, is only the tip of the iceberg. Often therapy services are covered by insurance, but co-pays, coinsurance, and deductibles can add up. Some providers do not accept insurance because the reimbursement is less than what individuals are willing to pay out of pocket. While we often speak of therapy as a time commitment, time translates into lost income, so a weekly commitment to take your child, on top of the out-of-pocket cost, can feel overwhelming. I would urge you not to write off the possibility before exploring your options; often there are resources available to help.

As a first step, I recommend you begin your search by speaking with your pediatrician, who should know the local options of care. Insurance companies can often help parents identify in-network providers where the costs will be less. Many states have early intervention programs, and schools employ social workers who can help connect families with resources should they not have insurance. School counselors can be another resource to help find appropriate support, and faith leaders are often invaluable resources in supporting members of their community in their times of need. The National Alliance on Mental Illness maintains a help line to connect families with local support specific to their need and circumstance. For urgent needs and crisis intervention, 9-8-8 has been recently established as the equivalent of 9-1-1 for emergency access to mental and behavioral health support. I've included other resources in the list at the end of the book.

Too often, families wait until mental health struggles reach crisis level before asking for help. This is understandable—as parents, we hope that with good parenting and time, issues might settle down or dissipate. Considerable strides have been made in recent years in acknowledging that mental health matters. Indeed, few things matter more to your child's well-being than their mental health. We know that many mental health disorders are rooted in neurobiology, an imbalance of neurotransmitters. But many parents still feel sad, hurt, or embarrassed that they aren't able to "fix" their children's mental health issues on their own. Additionally, sometimes anxiety and depression can have an insidious onset, where things slowly change over time. Parents are so close to the situation; they can adjust to this incremental worsening and consider it their child's baseline or normal state. It can be difficult for parents to know where to draw the line and decide to seek outside help.

With Sarah, the anxiety didn't come on quickly; certainly, if she had gone from racing into new experiences to becoming hesitant overnight, the change would have seemed concerning. But she had always been hesitant about new things, and slowly over time she became more so. At first, her tendency to repeatedly seek support from her parents seemed part of her personality and a healthy way of communicating what was on her mind. But her need for their comfort gradually increased and became more and more time intensive. When her mom looked back over a day or a week, she realized that a minimum of an hour a day was spent supporting Sarah's mental health. She would talk her daughter through small disagreements with her friends that invoked distress, help her double-check her schoolwork, and provide her reassurance after her interactions with others. After the parent-teacher conference, Mom took a step back and realized that for their family, "normal" meant that more time was devoted to Sarah's mental health than was spent with her sibling or doing things together as a family. The condition snuck up on the family, and it was now urgent for her to receive overdue care.

Children receive belated mental health support for other reasons too. Commonly, parents fear that pediatricians or psychiatrists may push medication as the only solution to a mental health concern. Please know that a full assessment is generally recommended before any treatment is offered for a mental health concern. This assessment is often eye-opening for families, as you learn more about your child's condition and what your options are. Best practice is for shared decision-making, where once an assessment is complete, a health-care provider offers ways to move forward with treatment. Depending on the circumstances, your care team may suggest several options, including therapy, medication, a combination, or monitoring your child's condition without immediate intervention. Mental health struggles may create feelings of vulnerability, but you retain your ability to decide what's best for you and your family.

Mental health providers generally do not have an agenda for the way you move forward. As much as some families may hesitate to consider psychoactive medication, other families may view the time commitment or cost of intensive therapy as inconceivable. Sometimes having options can be confusing or overwhelming, but it can also be a gift. You can know that multiple options exist to help your child, and whether or not you are interested now, you can learn about what medications may be options, why those are recommended, and what the advantages and disadvantages are to consider. Even if medication is strongly suggested, it is within your rights to say no and ask for alternatives.

Still, while some fear mental health medication, many adults maintain a preconceived notion that talk therapy cannot possibly solve their problems. However, hundreds of studies show that therapy is remarkably effective for a range of mental health challenges, with 50 percent experiencing improvement in eight sessions and 75 percent experiencing improvement from therapy alone.[7] This holds true for a large variety of diagnoses and age groups, and many imaging studies even demonstrate changes in the appearance of the brain consistent with the types of improvements seen by using medication. The hours of time in therapy and outside of therapy practicing new skills and thought patterns can provoke changes in your brain architecture and chemistry similar to the changes seen by psychoactive medication—which is evidence to support the validity of both treatment options.[8] Even those who believe in the need for therapy often have difficulty obtaining and paying for such services—a topic I'll revisit in Chapter 13.

As you consider therapy, numerous questions may arise. One of the first is: What type of provider is appropriate? Many professionals have credentials to provide therapy, including psychiatrists (medical doctors), psychologists (master's degrees or doctoral degrees in mental health), social workers (master's degrees or licenses), marriage and family therapists (training in couples and family counseling), and counselors (master's degrees or licenses). The training doesn't necessarily dictate who will be the best fit for your condition. As you decide how to move forward, if there is diagnostic uncertainty or a likely need for medication, starting with a psychiatrist makes sense. Otherwise, the best individual may be determined based on matching with someone who seems to have the most constructive professional relationship with your child.

Many therapists have specific scopes of practice, with expertise within certain age ranges and with certain diagnoses. It's important to ensure your child's condition is a good fit for their area of interest. Not all therapists offer all therapies, so if you are looking for someone to work with your seven-year-old about anxiety, someone who is more professionally focused on teenagers struggling with depression would not be the best fit. Because therapy is more intimate, the therapist's personality and working style matter more than with other specialists. Particularly when we're asking our child to engage in work that may feel uncomfortable or difficult, finding the right fit can make a big difference. The fit is so important that it's not uncommon to try a second or even a third provider to find a better fit. A provider you can afford is another important limitation, as we discussed above.

Unfortunately, in many communities and even within our own families, we can find individuals who are outdated in their understanding of mental health and carry negative or judgmental attitudes. You may be unlucky enough to experience this when you choose to share your diagnosis. Families can struggle to find the words to explain to others in their community what they are facing when a child is impaired by their sadness, anxiety, or other behavioral health challenges. But as you decide, don't forget to consider the potential benefits of being open about your challenge.

When a child has a physical health challenge, some communities rally with meal trains and offers of support. One of the biggest reasons we don't see this same support with mental health challenges is privacy. If you are able to be open about it, you may be pleasantly surprised by others who can empathize and help. Remember that nearly one in five children has a mental health concern, so there are other families in your children's class at school or in your neighborhood with similar experiences, even if you aren't sure who they are from the outside. Even if you don't have others reaching out to offer support, when you disclose diagnoses, it's also possible that you will help others following behind you to know it's okay to ask for help. Mental health concerns aren't the only challenges that lead families to feel stigmatized or isolated, and we worry about bullying and confronting ignorance. Parents struggle with these feelings and must help their children cultivate and maintain positive self-esteem and resilience. Later in the book, I'll provide practical suggestions for confronting these types of challenges.

Before you move on, consider:

- Does your child need behavioral health services they aren't getting?
- What are the main barriers to getting those services?

- If you have felt isolated or stigmatized because of mental health needs, what could you do to change your community for the better?

Working with Early Intervention Services and School-Based Support Teams

My complex-care practice at an academic medical institution involved working fifty hours or more a week and taking patient phone calls one out of every three nights. Though I loved my patients and my team, and I loved doing research and educating future pediatricians, I needed more time and energy to focus on my own growing family. I was not willing to abandon my professional goals, but I decided that moving my practice to a public school setting would allow me to have better boundaries. Something that helped me make this transition was knowing that school is where most children spend most of their time. The potential impact of appropriate school services on improving a child's quality of life is substantial.

Working within the New York City public school system meant I could have summers off and do shift work. No one would call me in the middle of the night or on weekends. Even so, in many ways going from a hospital setting to a school setting was a more difficult shift than I anticipated. I went from knowing everything about my one hundred patients to knowing next to nothing about the 120,000 children served by my district's schools. I learned a lot during that time, but one essential takeaway was that every school, even in the same district, in the same neighborhood, had a different way of doing things.

The school offices had the same paperwork, the same job titles filled, and supposedly the same processes, but the stakeholders—the people who you really needed to talk to when a child needed a specific type of support—were different in each scenario. Some principals took a more hands-on role and some secretaries took on leadership roles in delegating services. Each school had a cohesive process, but I found that parents need to learn how their child's school works in order to understand what you need to do to get your child the services they need.

Complexity of the system aside, sending a child to school while they face a challenge is often emotional. In her book *Raising a Rare Girl*, Heather Lanier summarizes how she attempted to navigate entrusting her special needs child to the local school. Her child was smaller than the other children and needed more support. She says, "You do three things. You prepare the school professionals as best you can. You tune your instincts keenly to their responses, sussing out whether they seem competent and respectful of your kid. And then if your instincts approve, you let go."

While I haven't navigated the process of sending a child with challenges to school as a parent, I can affirm that sending any child to school is stressful. There's separation anxiety at drop-off, fatigue and pent-up emotions that get dumped on the parent at pickup, and the new uncertainty of not knowing exactly what happened at school. Did your child drink enough water, eat enough food, or use the bathroom? Were your child's peers kind and inclusive? Did your child have meaningful engagement with the education provided? When your child is facing challenges, there is even more to worry about.

That said, school can be invaluable to both parent and child. The separation of your life from your child's life can help both of you to grow. Your child will grow and learn and have a space of their own. You will have more room in your life for your own concerns. And if your child has faced challenges, in some way the school community can offer even more benefits: special education services and occupational, speech, and physical therapy not provided through health insurance. Schools can offer teaching plans customized to your child and access to skilled professionals who often care for your child and provide you as a parent with coaching and daily support.

But it's not an easy transition, and when your children have challenges, the stakes feel higher. In practice it can be very difficult to sort out "I'm stressed about this transition" from "I don't trust my children's school." Teachers, similar to medical professionals, often pursue their career through a passion for helping children. This means that most of the time they share your goals and strive to work in the best interest of your child.

Teachers, therapists, and educational professionals are still only human, with their own strengths and weaknesses. Sometimes we don't know what we don't know. Just as in medicine, educational best practices evolve over time and some schools will be more up to speed and willing to try new things, while other schools may have a more traditional approach. The range of the quality of care schools can offer can be broad. The only way to know is to do the research.

As you approach decisions about school, be honest and up front about your child's needs. You'd much rather the school be the right fit than have your child struggle without appropriate support. As part of your research, ask other parents about their experiences with the school. Seek out community resources through social media or educational advocates and consultants.

Individuals with Disabilities Education Act

As you parent your child or children through challenges, it's important to be aware of one particular law, if you aren't already: the Individuals with Disabilities Education Act (IDEA). This law provides that all children with disabilities are entitled to a free and appropriate public education to meet their unique needs. The law provides protections at many levels: Parents must give consent before evaluation and before services are started. They have rights to input and for independent evaluations at the government's expense. The law emphasizes the need to keep children side by side with their peers in the least restrictive environment. There are provisions for mediation of conflicts and complaints. The way in which this law is interpreted varies, and local resources may be your best bet at helping understand how it applies to your family.

From 2019 to 2020, 7.3 million students aged three to twelve received special education services under IDEA.[9] This adds up to 14 percent of public school students, all of whom receive accommodations under a specific category. There are many categories of disabilities, including autism, visual or hearing impairment, deaf-blindness, emotional disturbance (which can include diagnoses such as depression or anxiety), intellectual disability, orthopedic impairment, specific learning disability, speech or language impairment, traumatic brain injury, multiple disabilities, and other health impairment (which could include diagnoses like ADHD).

Developmental delay is a category that can sometimes qualify for accommodations, though the definition and covered age range varies considerably by state. Nearly all children who struggle in school will qualify, but sometimes school choice or quantity or frequency of school services may vary depending on which category you qualify for. If you're unsure if your child's issues are covered or if your child is receiving services in the most appropriate category, please reach out to your school and to local advocacy groups.

It's important for parents to be organized in order to navigate the complexities of school services. While some conversations may seem like friendly ones about your child's school day, it's wise to remember that, on the other side, whether public, private, or parochial, the school is bound to rules and protocols. Make requests in writing, ensure all communications are marked with dates, and keep records and ask for written responses. If the school says no to an intervention you've requested, remember it may not be a decision based on your child but one based on their capacity to offer necessary support.

Lastly, as you have conversations with educators about interventions in educational considerations, I'd urge you to ask for the recommended interval for reevaluation. Most schools recommend reevaluation every two to three years, and it can take at least three months for educators to develop an educational plan. If you are used to thinking of medical interventions, where you see improvements in a few weeks, it can be disappointing but not unexpected to have to wait longer to know if educational interventions are effective. Be sure to have a realistic expectation from the beginning.

As you think through the support your child is getting at school, think of the following questions:

- Do you think your child is getting the support they need to thrive? If not, what changes could you make to support them?

Do you understand how the system works at your child's school to adjust the plan and communicate effectively? Would you benefit from more organization in your communications with school? I hope reviewing the systems where your child will receive care has been helpful. When you are helping your child through a challenge, sometimes the devil is in the details. If you don't take the medication, see the right specialist, understand your follow-up plan, or find the right behavioral and educational support, you may have more difficulty addressing your child's challenge. But another key component of your plan is understanding the big picture. In this chapter we focused on the specifics, but in the next we'll zoom out to understand the common patterns faced by families in your shoes.

CHAPTER 4

Understanding the Bigger Picture

Born preterm at twenty-four weeks, Manuel had almost every possible complication. He had an episode of bleeding in the brain, which led to hydrocephalus, or increased fluid retention in the brain, requiring multiple surgeries. This brain trauma led to recurrent seizures that couldn't be controlled despite many medications, and his preterm birth resulted in lung disease. Each time he had a respiratory illness, he was admitted to intensive care. His feeding and growth difficulties required many procedures and feeding by a central line infusion or a tube. Shortly after we finally found a feeding regimen that worked, he would have an infection of his hydrocephalus shunt, requiring further hospitalization, long-term antibiotics, and more surgery. Just when that infection was clear, his epilepsy would worsen and change, requiring extra testing and new medications.

By age two, this became a clear pattern for him. Whenever one of his health issues would improve or stabilize, something new would come up. When he was again admitted to the hospital intensive care unit with a respiratory illness, I spoke with Manuel's mother, who shared through tears that she was newly pregnant.

At the bottom of her distress was guilt that the new baby would take attention and family resources away from Manuel. She was worried that any slip in her vigilance might harm her son to whom she was so devoted. But something she said really resonated with me: "We just have to keep living our lives. I know with my son, it's going to continue to be like this, and I have to do my best for him without having his medical issues be the only thing in my life."

This mother's dedication to her son was impressive, but her ability to see this perspective amidst the chaos of back-to-back hospital stays really stuck with me. She had been able to remember who she and her husband were before Manuel's illnesses and connect with what their long-term goals were for their family amidst ongoing chronic trauma. She was, in many ways, brave to make this choice because it was important to her and her husband. Even though they didn't know how they would manage, they had faith they would figure it out.

Regardless of the size or severity of your struggle, because parents care so much about their children it's quite tempting to let the issue at hand take over. Sometimes this makes sense; in a crisis, devoting a lot of resources and attention short-term may pay off. But pausing to recognize the big picture is essential so you can consciously make a plan that makes sense for your whole family.

Identifying the Pattern

Challenges tend to fall into patterns, and the pattern can help you predict what's coming and choose a response intentionally. Manuel's mother had recognized the difficult pattern of her son's illness, which was crisis after crisis, slowly progressing, and getting worse.

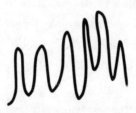

In the graphic above, imagine that time is on the bottom axis moving forward. The ups and downs illustrate the times when the child is doing well and then times when the child is experiencing more hardship generally. The hardships include more symptoms and difficulty due to the challenge, more appointments, and more disruption.

For Manuel's mother, it was unsustainable for the family to live in emergency mode all the time. She was in her late thirties and wanted to have more children. She knew putting that off indefinitely did not make sense for her. She worried that others would judge her for this choice, but all I saw was a woman who had the perspective and sophistication to see the bigger picture and remember that other goals and relationships mattered too.

Your challenge may be smaller, less disruptive, and more manageable. You may not be dealing with constant hospital visits; your child might have chronic environmental allergies that trigger asthma attacks that can be managed with an inhaler. Your life may seem like this illustration, with ups and downs of a smaller scale. Your child is basically all right, but every few weeks there is a period where he requires frequent albuterol, increased medication, or a doctor's visit, like this:

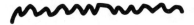

You may think, "Things are pretty good. I understand our challenge, we have a safety plan, and we try to avoid big crises." But it's important to be aware of how much energy, work, and stress you are putting in to achieve the result you are getting. Where would the baseline for your family's day-to-day life be if things were better?

This insight requires an intimate understanding of what happens in your child's life within your specific family *and* an awareness of what's medically possible and realistic. For some families in this situation, the daily stress of medication, monitoring symptoms, and stepping up therapy as needed might feel manageable. Maybe things could be a little better, but in a household where the parents have some flexibility in their schedules and the child's regular activities aren't too disrupted, maybe the baseline isn't too far away.

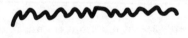

In this scenario, the wavy lines of good days and bad days reflect small swings, and the baseline of where things could possibly be is not far off.

For other families whose children have the same condition, their day-to-day experience may be much more difficult. They may be using nebulized medications that take ten minutes to administer and are dosed three times a day, and the child may resist vigorously each time, to the detriment of the relationship with parents. The commute to school may be slow and laborious and interrupted by coughing. The school nurse may seem to always be calling and sending the child home. The magnitude of the day-to-day normal is farther away from the baseline of where the family would live without the asthma and allergies. This may feel excessive even if you are doing everything right as a parent.

The doctor working with this particular family might check in about the child's asthma control to get some metrics—how many nights of sleep are interrupted and how many school days are missed—but even these metrics offer limited insights into what life is actually like. In this scenario, the ups and downs are still small, but the daily toll is larger, making this less acceptable to the family.

If the daily load is more than your family can handle, you can talk to your care team about the options you may have. You can discuss options with your team or do your own research to find what's medically possible. Unfortunately, I've seen so many families fall into a state of learned helplessness and miss these potential perspectives. I've heard families in this position say things like, "He just will never be able to run and play without his asthma acting up." Depending on the context of what's been tried, this is almost certainly incorrect. It can take a while to find the right therapy, but most children can achieve control of their asthma.

Only a Parent Can See

Facing any challenge can be traumatic, and facing challenges that impact your child even more so. Trauma, particularly when recurrent, can induce feelings of powerlessness. Some parents give up hope for improvement and just accept the status quo as their reality. Sometimes this instinct is helpful; you save your limited energy to power through and do what needs to be done. But this acceptance may prevent you from advocating for change.

Say a doctor is seeing both of these families in their clinic: one child has manageable asthma; the other does not. If both parents say, "Yes, managing asthma and allergies is a day-to-day thing, but it's not worse than before," the doctor will likely advise them to continue the current plan. But perhaps the second family, the one who feels it all is too much, has the perspective to say, "No, it's too much; it really isn't working." This may be all it takes to advocate for some other options.

Unfortunately, this is one way privilege leads children to receive different levels of care. A parent who has more education, more research, more time, or a more knowledgeable network may have this awareness, speak up, and advocate more than a parent who has less knowledge, less money, a less flexible job, a less knowledgeable network, or faces bias from a medical system.

When a parent does have the ability to advocate and ask for more help, the doctor can dig into the details of the situation and explain what the reasonable options are. Sometimes adjusting the medication—one that's less of a struggle to administer and more effective—might improve the family's everyday experience. Sometimes, a larger investigation is necessary. It is possible that the family has a dog that triggers the chronic allergies, which then triggers the asthma. The sad result could be parting with the dog—which would certainly lead to emotional turmoil—but it might make the family's day-to-day better in the long run.

Alternatively, they could consider weekly allergy shots, even though this intervention requires a lot of time and causes the child some discomfort. But, if the investment of five hours a week for six months leads to improvement of allergies and asthma in the long run, perhaps the time and cost are a better option—and the beloved family dog gets to stay.

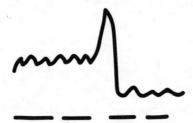

In this scenario, the big bump in the middle where things get worse may be one that you consciously choose—investing the time and energy to have a surgery that might lead to better disease control, for example.

Only a parent can know if this investment of time and energy in pursuit of better disease control makes sense. This line of thinking only works for a certain kind of problem, one that responds to intensive intervention. If your child needed allergy shots at the same frequency for the rest of their life, you might say, "Of course this wouldn't make sense." If your child has a long-term disability such as cerebral palsy, there may be times when intensive investment makes sense. The child may receive frequent therapy with the goal to reduce pain, reach a milestone, or recover from a procedure. But there may be other times when the priority is to keep things sustainable and do the therapy work only as needed to maintain your current status and prevent complications.

Managing Uncertainty about the Future

Other challenges, such as anxiety, can worsen over time without intervention. If a child perceives social interactions as threatening, she may engage socially less often. Over time she may have fewer social skills and perceive social settings as more intimidating and further withdraw. Parents can contribute to this spiral when they see their children feeling anxious and uncomfortable and make efforts to help. Sometimes parents inadvertently reinforce the idea that the child can't handle the situation independently or that the situation is scary.[1]

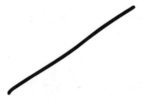

This is how we imagine a progressive disease or diagnosis that may worsen over time.

If you have a similar challenge that seems likely to get worse, the question is whether by intervening—spending more energy now by investing in finding the right resources to support you and your child in improving things—could alter the trajectory. You could read a parenting book about anxiety or seek out a therapist. Though these things may carry costs, and may even make things worse in the short-term, if you can alter the trajectory to improve things in the future, it may be well worth it.

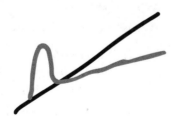

The lighter line imagines a scenario where you invest energy toward the goal of improving long-term control of a worsening or progressive process.

What makes these decisions especially difficult is uncertainty. While we approach many challenges with metrics and reports, challenges are inherently unique. The anxiety may worsen over the years as social situations become increasingly complex and your child becomes more focused on friendships, but it's not certain. Some children go through phases and develop and learn skills to improve things without intervention. There is no one exactly like your child and no family exactly like yours. So even the most experienced educator, therapist, or physician may be unable to predict what will happen going forward. You may have the sense that things may get worse, but they may get worse slowly, quickly, or not at all.

This uncertainty doesn't apply only to mental health or developmental challenges. Parents whose children face recurrent or progressive medical issues such as ear infections cope with similar uncertainty. Recurrent ear infections can lead to hearing damage, severe or resistant infections, interrupted sleep, impaired balance, and delayed motor milestones, and generally worsen quality of life. Doctors can guess which children will have more problems with their ears in the future based on their anatomy and their age. Often these doctors' opinions are quality educated guesses based on published studies and years of experience, but at the end of the day, it is still just a guess.

I'm sure most pediatricians have seen children who they thought had outgrown the propensity for ear infections catch some virus or become colonized with some bacteria and suddenly have ear infections worsen in severity and frequency. We also may know children who we thought for sure would worsen, who did not.

Knowing the reality of this uncertainty, approaching the question of surgical intervention for recurrent ear infection seems daunting. Some parents might choose to avoid surgery and their child might suffer more infections and end up having the surgery later on. Others might opt for surgery that may not have been necessary. No parent wants surgery and anesthesia for their child unless it's necessary, but doctors cannot know for sure when it is absolutely necessary. One of the most important parts of understanding the big picture is to see where there is certainty and where there is uncertainty. Sometimes your care team, in an effort to spare you stress, may not communicate with you the full extent of this uncertainty. But knowing this context can guide your decisions.

Example of a Care Map

Another way to imagine your big picture, particularly if your child has complex health-care needs, is to make a care map. Cristin Lind, the mother of a child with complex care needs, first created a care map in 2011 when trying to explain what life as a parent caregiver was like to a group of physicians at Boston Children's Hospital. In the middle she drew her son and her family in a circle. Then she drew a line out to other circles illustrating his biggest buckets of care needs—school, health, support, legal and financial, recreation, and information/advocacy. From each of these six circles she drew a line to each related individual. Around the health circle was the dentist, the primary care office, the pediatric subspecialists, and pharmacy and equipment vendors. Out of the school circle, lines connected the various therapists, educators, and transportation resources involved in her son's care.

Care mapping is a family-driven, person-centered process by which you understand what you are already doing. The circles and categories of a care map will vary based on a child's unique situation. Visually, it communicates both the big picture and the small details needed to support your child. When you make a care map, you have an opportunity to reflect on your situation, think of things that are missing or unknown, or see things that may surprise you. At the end, you have a resource that you can potentially share with team members or family and friends to help them understand your situation. A care map is a snapshot in time, but it can help you remember

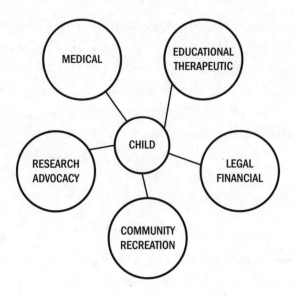

resources that you may be underutilizing or areas where you need to find more resources. If your child is gaining independence in navigating their own care, working on a care map together or comparing their version of a care map with yours can be a great tool to highlight gaps and differences.[2]

The Currency of Energy

One of the most useful takeaways from gaining a broader perspective about the challenge you face is that it can help you be more intentional and selective about how you spend your precious energy. Penny was a patient of mine with spastic quadriplegia; she was a wheelchair user, nonverbal, and relied on a breathing tube. She had significant functional limitations due to her disability, but for her family the day-to-day struggles were with her school.

The bus driver smoked cigarettes, which irritated Penny's lungs. After a fight with the school, he was replaced. But the new driver adhered rigidly to all rules, and if they were late or her wheelchair was not up-to-date with required service exams, she was not taken to school.

She had student aids who were insensitive and disrespectful. Penny's mother was never happy with the number of services allocated by the school's individualized educational plan for her daughter and was always upset that what was promised was not delivered. For example, the physical therapy plan specified goals about spending time in a stander, an alternative positioning device that would help her stand with appropriate support, reducing her pain due to muscle spasticity and preventing pressure ulcers from sitting in the same position in her wheelchair all day. The school aids would report to Mom that she wasn't moved out of the wheelchair all week, leaving Mom to feel confused, further eroding her trust in her daughter's care. She wanted the school to be helping her child, but most of her work with them was to ensure they did not reduce her daughter's quality of life.

Penny's mother was a lionhearted advocate for her daughter, always setting meetings, working with an advocate, and following up diligently. But it wasn't working. Eventually, I suggested she consider alternative schools. Perhaps the school wasn't able to meet her daughter's needs and another school could do better. While the mother had many times wished she could move her daughter out of there, she never envisioned it could be a reality. She was spending a ton of energy trying to make the current school work for Penny, but they lived in public housing and Mom worked full-time. She could not afford a specialized vehicle to transport her daughter or private school tuition.

With a massive effort from our social worker and educational advocates, Penny's mom channeled her energies into looking for alternative schools instead of trying to fix the current school. Nearly a year later, after many tours, numerous bureaucratic hoops, and a lawsuit, her daughter was transferred to a specialized school for children with brain injuries. The school had a much more ambitious plan for her daughter's care and the personnel to make it happen.

Penny's care was notably better. This changed two lives, as now her mother finally had peace of mind. She felt her daughter was safer and better attended to by professionals with the training and passion to advocate for her. This improvement in her circumstances was made possible because Mom redirected her energy. Instead of playing Whac-A-Mole with one school problem after another, she put her mind behind finding a better fit and did.

While in her scenario, her team was able to help her identify and redirect her energy, many families have to figure this out on their own. Take a moment to consider where you are putting your energy as you face your child's challenge:

- Are you being reactive or proactive?
- Are you getting good results from the amount of energy you are spending?
- Are you spending your energy in the best places?
- Are you allocating enough energy given the scale of the issue you face?

When Watchful Waiting Makes Sense

Some problems may resolve on their own, without much intervention. We see this often with speech delays. A father who is now fluent in multiple languages did not speak a word until he was nearly three years old. As a child, he wasn't offered much analysis or testing, and he was not seen by a speech therapist. He had two sons, and his eldest child didn't speak at all at eighteen months. Most children begin speaking around twelve months and acquire at least fifteen words by eighteen months. At this point, he was referred for interventions. The child saw an ear, nose, and throat specialist and an audiologist for a hearing test. Then he began thrice weekly speech therapy. Subsequently he began speaking after two and a half, just like his dad. Now he is an elementary honors student fluent in two languages.

When the next child came along, he also wasn't speaking at eighteen months. The father reflected on the big picture of their family's life. Thoughtfully, he questioned, "Do we really need to intervene?" I knew this family would have done anything for the benefit of their child—most parents would. But in the context of their family, knowing that father and older brother were both "late talkers," Dad was hesitant to put his child through all of the evaluations and therapy sessions if they might not be necessary.

Speech therapy has value and can help children in numerous ways, but any intervention takes away from other areas. The child may lose out on regular nap time or spend additional time restrained in the car, the parent misses work for the evaluation, or the visits risk exposure to viruses. And the speech therapy work, while often fun for the child, is not the same as play. The father wanted to understand how to balance his family's life with the need to support his son's development.

Many parents might shy away from discussing these decisions with the doctor—many might have taken the referral for the hearing test and early intervention services and decided later whether to use them. But I was so glad he asked, because it gave me the opportunity to help him find a middle road. I could explain why the hearing test was so important, and we could establish care with some trusted, experienced professionals and commit to close observation or a lesser frequency of services that was more sustainable for the family.

By remembering the big picture and communicating openly with the care team, this family was able to receive a more personalized plan of care that made sense to them and met the child's needs. Seeing your family's big picture can help you further improve a thoughtful plan.

We should acknowledge that we all only have so much energy. When we devote a lot of energy to a challenge, that energy is taken away from something else, whether it's your other children, your career, your self-care, your partner, or your friends. When approaching parenting without a challenge, there is always more you can do—such as more enrichment, more physical activity, more quality time, higher-nutrition meals, or extra sleep. But we know that more doesn't always make your experience as a child or a parent better.

In a medical context, more medications may mean more side effects, more doctor's visits may mean more unnecessary procedures or exposure to viruses, and extra imaging often leads to incidental findings that can cause harm. For parents, doing more on your child's behalf or overscheduling them can inhibit their opportunities for learning. Yet we all feel a lot of pressure to do more and sometimes propagate this cultural tendency. This tension has led to books about simple and minimal parenting, including my favorite, *Free-Range Kids* by Lenore Skenazy. In the book, Skenazy pushes back against the common narrative that children are incapable of contributing positively to their own development and argues that space and freedom to make mistakes enhance their growth. Encouraging independence has thankfully become mainstream.

But when parents approach challenges that threaten their child's well-being, this awareness is often lost. More is not always better when it comes to helping your child through a challenge. When we set the goals, we aim toward safety and health, but we also acknowledge that well-being often lives in the space between good enough and optimal. Knowing the big picture can help you make better decisions.

- You can be a good parent even if you do not take every opportunity to do *more*.
- You can be a good parent if you sometimes choose *yourself* over your child.
- You can be a good parent if you *disagree* with what the doctor or educator tells you is important.
- You can be a good parent if you *delay* something important for a valid reason.

Some things will not matter later on. If you are late a few times to school, or if your meals are slightly less nutritious than you might prefer, or it takes an extra two months to get a referral scheduled, in the big picture, it probably doesn't matter. Remembering this can help you feel a sense of peace when you drop a ball here or there while attending to some of the many important things on your plate.

Still, some things do matter. Living in crisis mode long-term can have a cost. I worry most about the demands on your well-being as a caregiver. Parents who are depressed or burnt-out suffer, and they may be less able to help their families. If you are always overstretched because you are pulled in a dozen different directions, and you yell at your kids more than you'd like or you miss the warning signs of deteriorating mental health of your "healthy" sibling, this matters. In my experience, caregiving parents who juggle several balls are more likely to drop one of the balls impacting their wellness than their child's wellness—though we know a family's well-being depends on everyone's health.

Using Your Energy Wisely

A family I worked with had a child, Leo, who struggled to adapt to nursery school. He was introverted and preferred to watch his classmates rather than jump into playing together. His teachers wondered if he might need developmental assessment and intervention because his participation in school was so restricted. He was hesitant to engage with new caregivers and teachers but was loving with those he was close to and he had a few friends with whom he played beautifully.

As I helped Leo's family make a plan for how to move forward, we had a few choices. We could view the school's assessment as intended, that what they saw at school suggested a larger developmental diagnosis or disability and proceed with evaluations and therapists. Or we could consider whether the child was the right fit for the school, given that his interactions outside of school hadn't concerned his other experienced coaches and caregivers. Perhaps another school would be a better fit? Or we could view his challenge as a simpler one—he hadn't yet connected with the students and made friends; perhaps we could help him make friends by having some small group playdates.

Depending on the nuance and exact circumstances of the situation, any of these might be reasonable ways to move forward, but the best path forward depends upon your bigger picture view of the challenge you are confronting. It may feel overwhelming to make this decision; it's important to your child's well-being and you lack certainty. But no matter which path you choose, reevaluation will help to ensure you've chosen correctly. In a few months it may be clear that allocating your energy toward more playdates isn't working and it's time to get a developmental specialist involved.

By seeing the big picture, you can pace yourself and make more sensible decisions. It's not always obvious whether your condition is a problem you should either live with or conquer. To further complicate matters, many conditions may be a mix of the two. Consider this child who has been slow to socially acclimate to preschool. Is the problem that our expectations of his behavior are too narrow? Not only do we expect him to express social behavior typical of his peers but to do it on our schedule. Or does he lack the skills to make friends and communicate? Perhaps addressing this need will help him to thrive and enrich his life? While it would be simpler if this were black and white, it takes a nuanced eye to decide whether our challenge is one to be "fixed," supplemented, and remediated or one where we learn to embrace our children's differences. Sometimes we need to correct a child's challenge, and sometimes we need to advocate for greater social acceptance of their differences.

The caregiving parent is the person in the best position to have the big picture and the deepest understanding of their child's lived experience. It's not an easy job to make decisions on our child's behalf, so in the next chapter I'll dive into some ways in which you can prepare yourself best to meet this responsibility. With the right preparation and seeing a zoomed-out view of what you face, you can select where you invest your energy and plan your life to fit your reality.

As we go on, take some time to consider where you are and what type of challenge you are facing. Imagine how you might look back at this time in six months or six years. If you are overwhelmed, this zoomed-out view of the problem can help. If you are struggling to see the big picture, speaking with your co-parent, family members, or other trusted friends can be invaluable. Sometimes when we are so close to a situation is when it's most difficult to see the bigger picture, but our loved ones can give us this necessary perspective.

Some questions to consider before we move on:

- Is my challenge big or small, predictable or unpredictable?
- How much day-to-day strain is associated with my challenge?
- Is this challenge long-term or short-term?
- Are things going to stay the same, or might they get better or worse?
- Can I affect the trajectory of what's to come?
- What's uncertain about this challenge?
- Have I communicated effectively with my care team, and do they understand what we are seeing at home?

PART II

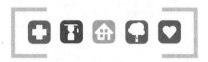

HOW TO TAKE ACTION

CHAPTER 5

Educating Yourself

Grayson had severe allergies to multiple foods—peanuts, tree nuts, eggs, and soy. His family lived with the daily restrictions and fear well known to families with children with life-threatening allergies. He was the oldest of four kids, and none of the others had food allergies; his mother blamed this on the evolving guidelines on the introduction of allergens. A couple years after his birth, the guidelines changed from recommending delayed introduction to early introduction of common allergens. Because of the timing of this change, she didn't expose Grayson to high-risk allergens until he was nearly two. In his first couple years of life, she kept him away from nuts and other common allergens because she was doing exactly what was recommended. But by the time his siblings came along the family had a pediatric allergist who shared the updated guidance and supported them through early and regular introduction of allergens.

Introducing allergens later in life could have been a factor in increasing Grayson's risk of food allergies, but it could also have been a coincidence. He may have been destined to be allergic no matter the timing of when he was given the foods. We'll never know, but his mom felt a fair amount of guilt and was reminded of it day in and day out as she dealt with protecting Grayson from accidental exposure in and out of the home—on top of the responsibility of raising four children.

Grayson's mother is a good friend of mine, and even as I reassured her that none of his allergies were her fault, she couldn't move past her feelings of guilt. To cope, she kept on top of researching Grayson's condition. If she had missed something previously, she was not going to permit this to happen again. This research led her to attend conferences about food allergies, subscribe to newsletters about food allergies, and consult multiple specialists. At times, I thought, "Maybe she should relax and trust her doctors."

But she was the first person I knew, despite my presence at an academic medical institution, to talk about oral desensitization protocols. At the time, the concept of inducing tolerance to allergens slowly over time by eating tiny amounts, then consistently increasing the amount of the food, was new. But she was spending time attending conferences and connecting with organizations advocating for novel treatments to pediatric allergies, and because of this work, she knew about this treatment option early. Once the clinical trial about oral induction of tolerance in our city opened, her child was enrolled. After hours and hours of frequent visits, Grayson built up his tolerance to nuts and tree nuts, and he seemed to outgrow the egg and soy allergies. While he had to maintain this tolerance by ingesting a lot of nuts, he can now eat all foods—though the family still carries his epinephrine as a precaution.

Increasingly, these oral immunotherapy techniques have become a standard of care, but my friend's efforts meant her son was one of the first to test them, and as a result, he benefited from the intervention years before he would have been able to access it through his primary allergist. Her diligence made a big difference for him, and the rest of the family.

While research may feel intimidating and imply deep dives into scientific databases and content accessible only to those with excessive time, money, or intellect, I would argue that research is for every parent. Research can include any method of learning more about what our child is facing and understanding our options. To me, searching online, reading educational websites, listening in on social media conversations relevant to your child's condition, and asking questions to other parents or members of your team all count as research.

Sometimes, parent research leads to direct benefit. Children can gain access to new technology, new referrals, or new medications that will improve their quality of life. Families facing challenges may find the right school, an appropriate caretaker or therapist, or a great summer camp that will help their child thrive. Research can often lead to smaller wins, too. Many families with prescription medications have large co-pays but can often find alternative medications or discounts from resources like GoodRx, Blink Health, Optum Perks, SingleCare, and other pharmacy discount programs from retailers like Walgreens, Walmart, Costco, and Amazon Prime.

But for some, maybe even most conditions, the benefits of research will be less tangible. You may not change your behavior or find better resources. In these situations, often you still benefit. You may gain context and a more nuanced understanding of what you face. You may confirm the information shared by your care team enhancing your trust in their advice. Research can connect you with other families who share your experiences and questions, helping to make you feel less alone. Research can lead you to gain confidence and comfort.

However, as with Grayson's mom, research can start to take over one's life, particularly when it's motivated by guilt or fear. Determining what is most relevant for your family can feel overwhelming. Even as a pediatrician, my research has sometimes led me down a search engine–enabled rabbit hole and made me feel nervous about concerns that weren't really important to my family. As with any other part of our life, we can go overboard on a good thing. Too much research can lead to wasted time, unease, or distrust. How can we gain the potential benefits of research while minimizing these costs? This chapter will focus on picking the best sources to trust and asking the right questions to get the answers you need.

Research: Make the Most of the Doctor

My patient Ben had been a sound sleeper for two years, but as he approached his third birthday, he started to backslide. He'd sleep for a few hours at the beginning of the night, and then he'd wake suddenly, writhing around in the bed scratching himself. He couldn't get the rest he needed, and as a result, he was fussy, tired, and less playful during the day.

Ben had eczema in the past, but it had never been so severe. Though the family had searched online and purchased some new products, Ben had developed a worsening case of chronic eczema, and it was causing his skin to bleed and scab. This wasn't just a problem for his own sleep; his entire family was exhausted and miserable. They came to me, eager for a solution. I discussed all the common causes of eczema—dry skin, environmental exposures, and allergies—and ways to adjust his environment to help, but their eyes glazed over until I mentioned a prescription. They were not in a place where they had the time or energy to learn—none of them had slept in weeks.

A few weeks later, they came back for a follow-up visit in a better place; Ben's skin was better, and the cream had helped, but when they stopped using it, they began to see the eczema come back. They had heard some of my advice at the last visit but lacked clarity on what they needed to do differently to keep the skin healthy. They changed Ben's bathing schedule, decreased the use of fragrant soap and detergent, and tripled the amount of cream and nonmedicated ointment used to promote skin hydration. This time, I felt confident that they heard the information I offered, and I thought that if the eczema did recur, they would know there were more interventions to consider and discuss.

I share this real-world story because it's important to remember that you can't learn everything you need to know about managing a chronic condition in one short visit with a doctor—even if your doctor talks quickly and you take notes. Often when you come looking for help or a short-term solution, the main information offered and heard is the plan.

You might have been in this situation with your child's treating professional. The plan offers you a solution and gives you action items to manage. The plan delivers a sense of the implications of a problem and helps answer the most pressing question: What do I do differently this week and next week?

However, it's hard to focus on a preventive plan when you have an immediate problem that needs to be addressed. Earlier I spoke about follow-up visits, and how sometimes they may not be a good use of time. It's easy for parents like Ben's to assume that as a doctor I offered a bad plan—when his skin got worse again, it was likely my fault. But at least I was able to communicate enough of the big picture for them to know there was more we could try.

Ben's parents chose to lean on the treating doctor to learn about and research his condition, and often that's a great strategy. Parenting a child through a medical challenge is hard, and while you can learn a lot online or through talking to other parents, your doctor offers curated information targeted specifically to your child with your unique living circumstances, medical history, and family history.

Time spent learning about the root cause of your child's condition is essential. Understanding the diagnosis will empower you to choose the best plan, but remember that your treating team is a great place to begin your search for information. Before you start researching specific treatment options or the best providers to manage the condition, first consider the fundamental question: Why are you facing what you are facing? Answering this question is not always solution oriented; you cannot always "fix" the cause of your child's challenge, nor do you always want to if their condition—disability, genetics, or diagnosis—is fundamentally part of who they are, but understanding the root cause will help guide your next steps forward.

In Ben's case, with his eczema, it was important for his parents to understand that the integrity of the skin and immediate environment would affect the severity of the condition. Changing his skin-care routine made it possible for his parents to address the root cause and

manage the condition with less medication. For another condition, perhaps a mood disorder like depression, it's unlikely you could control the
symptoms with one behavior change, because depression is inherently
too complex.

You can't always pinpoint the cause of a condition—usually it's some
combination of genetics, environment, and bad luck. But you can come
to understand what is happening to your child. Researching depression
can still help you learn that there are some behaviors that may have an
impact—adequate sleep, physical activity, and connection. But you'll
also learn that depression has a biochemical basis with structural and
functional changes in the brain. This knowledge may lead you to implement some helpful lifestyle changes for your child but retain the perspective that a medication may be necessary. This information can help you
to locate and select an appropriate care team.

As a conscious and engaged parent, the idea of learning more about
your child's condition might seem obvious. Of course, you'd take the
time to read up on the condition and gain important knowledge to aid
in their care. But I can tell you that for most people, it can be deceptively
difficult to find useful information on your own. When you are facing
a challenge, often there is an overwhelming quantity of information to
take in and so much content of variable quality.

The best place to start is to talk to your child's doctor. They are there
to support your family, and you should take advantage of them as a
resource. If you are given a diagnosis, you should be sure you understand
it. Ask questions.

Some questions you might ask:

- Will this go away?
- Why did this happen?
- Is there something I could have done to prevent it?
- How big of a deal is this?
- What is the urgency of addressing this issue?
- What happens if we do nothing to address this?

- What is likely to happen in the short-term and long-term?
- Do I need to change things at home or school in the short-term or long-term?
- Are other problems associated with this condition that I should look out for?
- Is this a very well understood condition with a clear plan, or is this an area where professionals disagree about the best plan?
- How will we decide on the right plan?
- Where should I go to learn more?

If you have been facing your challenge for a longer period of time, you might already feel like an expert, but there is always more to learn. The best source for your child's condition will vary, but a goal should be to have curated resources to help you understand your child's health. If your child has a condition supported by an advocacy organization, this is often a place to start. With my own health, I've been in a national research study about Wilms' tumor survivorship for nearly my entire life. When I became involved with the study at my doctor's encouragement, I was automatically subscribed to the advocacy organization and their newsletter. The newsletter contained more relevant information for me than nearly any other source.

When your child's condition fits well within an advocacy organization, that's a great place to look for information that is relevant to your family. In addition to informational websites, social media feeds, and podcasts, often these organizations offer support groups and opportunities to connect with other parents. Social media groups can help with this too; when new articles that are relevant come out, you may be more likely to hear about them from a group with shared concerns.

If your child's condition is rare or doesn't fit a specific organization well, identifying a scientific or educational leader in the field of interest can help. You could subscribe to their newsletter, attend their conferences or talks, or follow them on social media to get a curated take on what's relevant. In some circumstances, it may be helpful to place a search alert within your search engine of choice to alert you of news articles about the condition.

Parents can shift their mindset from being overwhelmed to staying curious. New treatments will come out and new studies will cause prior treatments to go out of favor. As a caregiving parent, you will find that you can always learn more—about what the diagnosis means for your child now or what it will mean, or a new way to process and understand why it happened in the first place.

Keep in mind, you aren't solely responsible for following updates in studies and treatment protocols. Part of the point of follow-up visits is to allow your doctor to review your plan of care and consider if the approach should change based on how your child is doing or how the body of knowledge about the condition has evolved.

Research Can Lead to Better Care

Consider Denise, a child who has been exhibiting worsening behavioral outbursts and poor sleep over the past few months. When her grandmother, her primary caregiver, takes her to the doctor, she receives a diagnosis of ear infection and is prescribed antibiotics, but despite treatment, the original complaints continue: behavioral outbursts and poor sleep. After a few weeks, the grandmother hires a sleep consultant out of frustration. After applying some of the consultant's tips, there is some mild improvement in the quantity of sleep, but the behavior problems continue.

Eventually at a teacher conference, Denise's preschool teacher brings up her propensity to mouth breathe and asks if the grandmother has ever talked to her pediatrician about sleep apnea. After this, the grandmother sets up an appointment and gets a referral for a sleep study. Then she learns, finally, nearly a year into this struggle, that the difficulties Denise has faced are likely due to sleep apnea and are fixable with a surgery to remove the tonsils and adenoids.

Was the diagnosis of an ear infection wrong? If she had fever and a bulging infection behind her ear, no. But it was incomplete. Perhaps if the pediatrician and caregiver had discussed Denise's broader medical history, the conversation would have revealed her loud snoring over a period of months. If the snoring was mentioned, the doctor might have discovered underlying sleep apnea earlier. The ear infection is related—likely the tonsils and adenoids led to poor drainage of the inner ear—but treating the infection did not help the root cause. Ideally, a thorough doctor would screen for sleep apnea, ask the right questions to get a thorough history, and provide more comprehensive care, rather than putting this burden on the caregiver.

But often the presenting questions, concerns, and appearance of the child drive the diagnosis and plan and in the real world, and things do fall through the cracks. Learning more about behavior outbursts and poor sleep might have led to a faster diagnosis for this family. The grandmother could have read books or articles on behavior or children's sleep, many of which bring up obstructive sleep apnea. If she showed up to that first appointment asking if snoring could be contributing to the behavior problems or focused on the longer-term duration of symptoms, maybe the referral for a sleep study would have been made months earlier.

Though undoubtedly this reflects problems with our health-care system—it should not depend so much on your advocacy—being a knowledgeable patient can get you better care. Doing research on your child's condition will help you ask better questions and emphasize the parts of your child's story that are most important.

Next Steps in Due Diligence

Let's assume you start your journey by asking all of the above questions. What do you do next? That varies, depending on the circumstances. Perhaps your child's school or childcare center raises a concern. Approaching your pediatrician, as we discussed above, is often the best next step.

Your pediatrician can help you put this concern in the context of your child's big picture and may offer different resources. You might be thinking, "But wait, my pediatrician isn't an educational expert." They may not be, but they are a great resource for pediatric health, and may be able to see issues that don't occur to an educational team.

Let's consider this issue through the lens of a common example. Your child's school has informed you they suspect your daughter has dyslexia. When you consult your pediatrician about this, they may ask questions about her mental health, since children with dyslexia are known to have a higher likelihood of attention deficit hyperactivity disorder (ADHD). Sometimes children with this diagnosis can have trouble coping with the stress of learning in a different way, such that they develop secondary struggles with self-esteem or mood. Your pediatrician might perform or recommend an eye exam to check that the issue isn't physiological; perhaps your child has vision issues and doesn't have dyslexia at all. This is research. It gets added to your knowledge bank so that you can put together the best care plan for your child.

As much as a physician's input is helpful, it's also a good idea to take concerns from the pediatrician to your school and childcare team. These professionals spend a lot of time with your child and know typical development well. They can often add more information and an important perspective to help you arrive at the correct diagnosis. Maybe they have seen other symptoms occurring at school and have not yet informed you. Maybe they have wondered if this was an issue and wanted to discuss it with you. Perhaps they think your doctor is wrong because they have observed evidence to the contrary. Whatever you learn may help your child. Once a treatment plan is started, the school should be informed so they can monitor your child's progress.

When Information Is Misinformation

My friend, a scientist (this fact will be important), had a daughter who experienced a stroke while in utero during her pregnancy. After her daughter's birth, the newborn was diagnosed with cerebral palsy. Amid her postpartum haze, my friend tried to learn as much as she could about neonatal stroke and the related challenges to prepare for parenting a child with a disability. She found articles about strokes and cerebral palsy leading to weakness and coordination difficulties. She learned a lot about the nutrition and developmental difficulties and risk of seizures her daughter might have. After she consumed a lot of content from big reputable websites, she continued to seek more information and joined several online groups for parents of kids who had experienced stroke.

In these groups she read about stem cell infusions as a therapy option for cerebral palsy. She found a few small clinical trials using stem cells to heal the damaged brain and spinal tissue of cerebral palsy patients. However, she also encountered nonmedical providers promising to "cure" her daughter's cerebral palsy with ten-thousand-dollar treatments not covered by insurance or done in conjunction with major medical centers. As she dove deeper, she noticed these websites promising a "cure" were using fear-based marketing techniques. The sites used threatening language, telling parents, "If you don't do this, your child will suffer." These websites featured many convincing testimonials and suggested that she was unwise to trust the advice from her physician. She was drawn into the promise of a cure and felt emotional and confused about what to do. In the end, she finally dismissed the entire idea because, as she put it, her "rational brain" spoke up. She would continue to follow the research and ask her daughter's team for updates on possible treatments, but not try something still investigational outside of a monitored and ethically reviewed clinical research trial.

In many ways, her experience reflects the most dangerous sort of misinformation. Medicine does involve a gray area; progress is always being made and early research is promising, but clinical research does take time. Without completing the studies and seeing the final results, we can't know the safest and best choice for a child, especially when potential treatments are invasive. In the meantime, enterprising individuals will prey on desperate parents, guilt-tripping them into making an expensive and potentially dangerous decision.

The internet is a great equalizer, and search engines have changed the world as we know it. We parents have so much information at our fingertips, and it's important to apply critical thinking skills when we go online. We all need to be mindful that the algorithms that drive search engines heavily rely on popularity and technical website factors that correlate with site reliability. We can't always count on this to present the most valuable, accurate information.

A search for one of the most common medications used for children's constipation, polyethylene glycol (Miralax), will lead you down a rabbit hole of misinformation. The top-ranked articles tend to have frightening claims on the dangers of the medication. Much of the content shown represents opinion, not fact, and is ranked prominently simply because of click frequency. Scary articles often provoke a response that promotes their ranking in search engine algorithms. Other content may be sponsored by competing products. As you do your research, how do you know which sources to trust? Unfortunately, it's not easy.

I suggest you start with the recommended resources from your diagnostic team. But you may want other additional sources—often families feel that doctors have bias due to the pharmaceutical industry or due to inertia and the relatively slow change to practice when newer and better treatments emerge. As you expand to other sources, you should develop a method by which you evaluate your content. If you can answer these three main questions—who wrote this? when? and can it be corroborated with other sources?—you'll be off to a good start ensuring its legitimacy.[1]

- **Who is the author?** Do they have a conflict of interest in presenting this information? Does the author have credibility? Do you agree with other parts of their content? Are their sources referenced? Is this someone's opinion or is the advice based on research?

- **When was the article written?** Is the information current or outdated?
- **Can you corroborate?** Are there other sources that agree? If you can only find one person concerned about something, there may be a reason no one else seems concerned.

The Benefits of Social Networks—On- and Offline

No two families travel the same path, but witnessing another family's experience may help you too. By definition, doctors and teachers center their assessment and plan on what they observe in the clinic or at school, not what happens at home. Your friends and your child's peers share the context of your broader life. Other family members, colleagues, and support-network members can be especially useful.

Andy was born after a particularly difficult pregnancy, one complicated by infection with cytomegalovirus, one of the viruses that causes infectious mononucleosis, also known as "mono." As a result of his mother's infection, Andy had viral meningitis while in utero. He was then born preterm, underweight, and with a neurological injury. His first year of life had been spent mostly in the hospital fighting respiratory infections and attempting to find a feeding program he would tolerate. Now three years old, he was more stable, but due to his brain injury, his development had stalled around the four-month milestones, he could not sit without support, and often had difficulty tolerating his oral secretions.

Andy's mother faced several barriers to care. She was young and lived in poverty in the Bronx. The only housing available to her was a family shelter, and she had literacy limitations and terrible insurance. Things that are simple for many were difficult for her. She had inadequate access to transportation and childcare; picking up a prescription refill or coming to an appointment were real hardships.

When Andy started preschool, his mother was quick to take advantage of the respite this childcare offered—she could use that time to learn about his condition, follow up with his care providers, and discuss his diagnosis with other parents. For the first time, Andy and his mother were part of a community of similarly abled children and families. She was savvy enough to observe his classmates in detail, asking their parents and caregivers questions and learning from them. She also learned a lot from the educators and therapists involved in his care at school.

She came back to my office, with increasing confidence and a long list of questions. She had ideas for improving his care. She had seen a collapsible wheelchair that was more practical for their life in the Bronx. She had heard that a specific brand of stander (a machine designed to support a child with weakness standing upright) was easier to use than the one they had been given. She had learned about blenderized diets—in which whole foods are blended and delivered by feeding tube rather than using prepackaged formulas—and wanted to give it a try.

Her son's new school had broadened her awareness of what was possible and provided her with a community of individuals to learn from. While the logistics of getting him to school were complex, and often it was frustrating when other families seemed to have it better or easier, these personal connections she made at school showed her different ways that life could look for a child with disabilities. These new relationships provided her family with immediate, tangible benefits, and connecting with others outside her home more regularly notably lightened her mood.

In the previous section, I suggested you consult both your child's pediatrician and school system; Andy's situation reminds us that connecting with other families can help too. While I, as a physician, do my best to anticipate needs and do research on behalf of my patients, there are limits to my ability to assist. At the time I was treating Andy, all of my patients were on public assistance and as a result, I hadn't seen the sort of equipment that was available with "good" insurance. I had never been to his home to see his equipment in action. I made assumptions about what would be the easiest to feed him for a family on a tight budget. All this to say, the school community helped this family in a way I couldn't.

Other parents can be an invaluable resource. You can benefit from talking to parents who are facing similar barriers to care and dealing with similar challenges day to day. Side by side, parents can imagine other possibilities for their children and better their approaches. Once parents learn about these opportunities, they can ask for support from their care team in making them happen.

The underestimated benefit of these peer supports is connection. Even with all the data and advice available to you, just speaking with another human who has been in your shoes can be more helpful than a Google search. Other parents can be especially helpful if your child has been diagnosed with something unfamiliar to you.

If you're having trouble finding someone or a group of people to connect with, you can ask your care team to connect you with another family. They may be able to select someone who is particularly a good fit. These local partnerships can be invaluable, because inevitably there will be a pharmacy, school, therapist, babysitter, or camp that comes up as a great resource. Many families who provide this advice and mentorship find the experience fulfilling as well.

If your child has been diagnosed with anything from ADHD to cancer, it's very likely you have turned to social media for connection, support, and advice. As a cancer survivor and a parent, I found great resources online that helped in a way my family and friends could not. Online support groups can filter and curate the news and relevant research. By learning what other people are asking about, you can anticipate things that may not have been on your radar. If you are facing something uncommon or you live in a rural area, social media can bring you together with other parents you might never have had the opportunity to meet.

Beyond that, learning from others' lived experience is one of the most valuable kinds of research; but remember, it is by nature anecdotal.

In the scientific method, we try to base our decisions on larger groups because we know how much variation occurs naturally. An individual's experience will become their truth and will not necessarily be *your* destiny. Two individuals with the same diagnosis can travel different paths. Grounding the experience of others in the bigger picture is important.

It's also important to be mindful when interacting with these groups, as some people can have bias. All of our experiences color how we see the world. If my child has moderate asthma and I seek support in a caregiver chat room, I may encounter a parent of a child with severe asthma. She may give me advice based on her experience that may or may not apply to my child. She may say, for example, that the medication my doctor recommended is no good—it did not help her child, and he needed a stronger one. But this advice is out of context; she doesn't have all the information my doctor had about my child's condition when she recommended that drug. This well-intentioned advice may be incorrect for my child and undermine my confidence. The loudest and most engaged participants often have been through traumatic experiences themselves. You can learn from these experiences, but some of the judgments they make can be flawed, especially when they don't know your story and you don't fully know theirs. Even if their doctor didn't help or the typical treatments didn't work for them, it doesn't mean your child will necessarily have the same experience.

As we discussed at the beginning of the chapter, be wary of what you find online. The larger social media groups often have group dynamics and politics in play. Some members may have an agenda such as selling a product targeted at other parents. Those who have had particularly difficult experiences might be overrepresented, as those who have not had trouble may spend less time engaging online. Some may see things from a different perspective than you—perhaps they have more or less resources available or other goals for their children. As you engage in these groups, check in with yourself to see if you are finding the benefit exceeds the confusion or if it's adding stress, and be selective.

Is the Research Ever Complete?

Certain aspects of parenting have become predictable rabbit holes. When you are expecting your first baby and trying to determine what sort of mattress is safe, you can spend weeks learning more about crib mattresses than you ever wanted to know. You may do the same when it's time to introduce solid foods or when approaching potty training—and the amount of available information and opinions is mind-boggling.

When your child is facing a challenge, there are even more opportunities for this to happen—and they are often higher stakes. You can spend hours researching every doctor or therapist you work with. You can go back and forth and debate every medication and treatment. Curating the information can take just as much time and energy as reading and processing the information. You can quickly become overwhelmed by the quantity of information out there, and you may have fewer social supports who can relate or guide you to the answers you seek.

At some point, the amount of research you've done has to be enough. And, at that point, the benefit of continued research diminishes. Some topics warrant more research than others—perhaps if your child is going to have a major surgery, or you are deciding on a topic that will have an everyday impact on quality of life, such as which school to attend. When you do research, you may feel like your anxiety is being quelled by the feeling of preparedness you gain, but this can backfire. Excessive time spent researching may take away from other valued activities—connecting with loved ones and spending time on things you enjoy. If you look hard enough, you will always be able to find someone who disagrees with your medical plan, and sometimes focusing on this will sow doubt or unease.

Parents often feel the drive to do the most research when facing the toughest decisions. Imagine you are expecting a baby who has been diagnosed in utero with congenital heart disease. As you try to pick where you will deliver and which pediatric cardiology team will support your child, you are forced to make a very difficult decision. On the one hand, the delivery and subsequent hospital stay and surgery required will be stressful. Being close to home, supported by family and friends, and being able to be there for your other children may help make that time better. However, you also want to have the most qualified surgeons and cardiologists involved in your case. So, you may prefer to travel to make sure the baby has access to the best team. But the cost and inconvenience of this will be immense. Not only will it complicate things in the short-term, but you'll have likely have to travel back for follow-ups longer term. And in the end, depending on how the baby does after delivery, it may not prove necessary to have emergency surgery at all.

When facing a decision like this, one with no clear answer, you can end up circling and feeling more and more anxious about the situation. There are advantages and disadvantages to each choice. While your choices aren't equal, your choices are similar in caliber. Each have considerable benefits and drawbacks. No amount of research can tell you which decision would be best for your family, nor can it tell you exactly what will happen to your family. What research can do for you is provide you with peace of mind that you have done your due diligence and done your best to obtain information to help you make the best decision you can.

I recommend that parents try to find a happy medium: do some research and store away some nuggets of information, but establish limits. To avoid overdoing it, keep a specific goal in mind when you do your research—perhaps during a sitting you'll focus only on researching specialists or learning about the side effects of a medication. Then avoid getting sidetracked. Monitor how much time you spend, especially on social media. If you find yourself spending an hour or more, think critically if it's time well spent. This will help you budget your time and pick your priorities.

Check in with the emotions related to the reading you're doing. Is more research adding to your stress or undermining your confidence? If you encounter upsetting or confusing information, have a plan to bring the information back to some of the professionals on your team before you worry too much. Your doctor, educator, or mental health professional may not be able to answer all of your questions, but he or she can hopefully address the ones most important to you and refer you to more reliable sources. You can always go back and ask more questions.

If your family or your team start to seem annoyed by your research, rather than getting defensive, approach the situation with curiosity. You can look to the person who is expressing annoyance—are they truly upset with you or frustrated they can't help you better? Sometimes this is a sign you are asking the wrong person for help or reassurance, or you could be asking the wrong questions. You can also look inward. Sometimes when others express concern for your behavior it's because your behavior is problematic. Excessive researching or worrying about the worst, especially if it's a pattern, could be a symptom that you are suffering from intrusive anxiety. While worry can be a normal feeling when facing a difficult challenge, when it begins to cause this sort of difficulty, sometimes anxiety warrants intervention such as therapy or medication to promote your coping. Or perhaps you can simply take a pause, and remember you are doing the best you can for your child and that you need to care for yourself too. The research will always be there.

In this chapter, we've discussed how research can include more than scholarly pursuits. Conversations you have with your child's doctor and other stakeholders in your child's care or with other caregiving parents are often more helpful than the latest peer-reviewed study, as the advice comes from those who know your child. While more knowledge can enable you to be a better advocate for your child, as with many things it's a balance, and excessive research can worsen unease and be a sign of anxiety. For many, reading a book (like this one!) can feel more manageable than searching online.

Building your knowledge base is just one of the many skills that can help you in your advanced parenting journey. In the next chapter we'll discuss how time management, communication, organization skills, and other tools can help make your life easier. But before we move forward, consider:

- Have you done all due diligence about what you are facing?
- Are any of your sources less than fully reliable?
- Is social media helping more than it's hurting you?
- There's a spectrum of parents—those who underinvest in research and those who overdo it. Where do you think you lie?

CHAPTER 6

Tools, Skills, and Tips to Build You Up

My daughter was born six weeks early, and when I took her for routine visits to the pediatrician, we both noticed she had a side preference. While many parents might think a side preference is typical—after all, I'm right-handed—in infants, only looking in one direction or using one side more than the other can be a sign a child needs more developmental assessment and support. So, we agreed to refer her to early intervention. Though I wasn't too concerned, I was aware her sidedness might lead to difficulty feeding, an abnormal head shape, or developmental delays.

We got the referral from the pediatrician and we called to schedule an appointment, but we were put on a waitlist. There was paperwork to be completed and faxed, and administrative obstacles along the way. One agency had to process the request; another did the intake evaluation. Prior to the evaluation, our pediatrician had to complete a form and submit it by fax. This all took a few weeks, and when my daughter was finally evaluated, she was eligible for services due to her asymmetry, but before those services could start, we had to find yet another agency that had availability to work with her—and we had to have a consultation meeting to discuss her case.

Now I can very much appreciate how those who designed the system might have thought having a consultation meeting would be helpful. We could discuss the findings of the evaluations, make a plan, and I could get answers to my questions. But as a parent, every additional step in the process, every meeting, has a cost. At this point I had already invested fifteen hours and waited three months for my daughter's therapy. One more consultation in person meant I'd have to take more time off work, and there'd be lost time in the commutes to the agency office. Instead, I wanted the meeting to occur by phone.

I simply couldn't justify taking a day off work to go across town in the middle of the day and sit with these therapists when everything could have been discussed remotely. If I was going to take a day off work, it would be to enjoy my free time with my child. So, when I said I was unable to attend the meeting, I was told that my child would not be eligible for services.

I knew better than to accept this. I pushed back and escalated the matter to the supervisor level. They admitted that the real reason they couldn't do the meeting as a conference call was because they needed the physical paper with my signature on it. A fax or a scan would be insufficient. We got through all of this, and she had her first physical therapy appointment nearly four months after being referred for early intervention. Though she would not let the therapist within six feet of her without wailing (she had met the developmental milestone for detecting strangers early!), we both agreed it was clear—she no longer showed any signs of the side preference that led us to start the process. The asymmetry was most likely due to her prematurity, and she had outgrown it on her own.

This is a perfect example of the types of roadblocks parents facing challenges encounter every day. Though many systems are created to serve families' needs, the cumulative weight of these burdens on families is underestimated. Each step along the process—being asked to get a form from my doctor, asked to miss work, asked to schedule multiple meetings with different stakeholders, and asked to complete paperwork—carries a cost, and the time and energy required quickly adds up. To add another layer to this, from a public health perspective, every additional step and barrier leads to more disparate outcomes based on language, education, and privilege.

As parents, so much of our labor is unseen: meal planning, finding childcare, enrolling in and preparing for school, stocking the right size clothing, and procuring developmentally appropriate toys and books. But caregiving parents often have even more labor—scheduling appointments and services, researching treatment options, dealing with insurance and reimbursement, educating others, advocating for their child's inclusion, and the emotional work of worrying.

As numerous as the challenges are, I know that I have so much privilege. I have reliable wireless internet, plenty of cell phone minutes, a stable mailing address, access to a fax machine, and fluency in written and spoken English and medical jargon. On top of this, I know my rights, and I'm not intimidated or dissuaded when I am told this is the only way my child can get help. Additionally, I have trust in the service providers and faith in the process as necessary. But privilege and preparation don't eliminate the time tax.

One of the reasons I became a pediatrician was because children have parents as built-in advocates. During medical school, when I saw adult patients in the clinic, I would advise medication or imaging and adults might not get it done. At the follow-up visits, they would shrug and admit it wasn't a priority. But when I saw children, I found that the parents were often on it, either taking on the responsibility for following my recommendations or holding the child accountable for doing so.

However, there are limits to what a parent can take on—even an exceptionally caring and thoughtful parent is still human. The inefficiency and difficulty of the medical system will wear you down. When you are taking care of your whole family and a child facing a challenge on top of everything, potentially for years, there will be times when you just lose the steam and motivation to face these hurdles. The work of caregiving feels never-ending. In fact, one of the most popular books on caregiving for people with Alzheimer's disease and other dementias, *The 36-Hour Day* by Nancy Mace and Peter Rabins, is titled such because caring for another person doesn't reduce the amount of time you need to spend on yourself.

So, we have to find strategies to make the work of caregiving in tandem with parenting more manageable. Families can learn about some of these tools from popular books, like Emily Oster's *The Family Firm* and Bruce Feiler's *The Secrets of Happy Families*, in which the authors take inspiration from corporate settings and apply best practices to family life. The thought here is that your home functions like a miniature business—it's a group of people dedicated to a shared purpose and outcome. We can learn from how companies run businesses to run our homes optimally.

This analogy may not resonate with everyone. Many of us think of words like *love*, *comfort*, and *connection* when we think of family life, rather than words like *efficiency*, *productivity*, and *return on investment*. However, if we look at family life with a bit more objectivity and distance than normal, we may be more open to consider change. While your home may contain the people you love the most, there are still day-to-day processes that have to happen—meals prepared, laundry done, appointments made, prescriptions filled. When we manage these processes and workflows optimally, by being more organized or efficient, by delegating more or improving communication, we can decrease our stress levels and potentially increase the energy left over for the relationships and love that is so important to us. The tips, tricks, and skills covered in this chapter will primarily focus on managing the work of running your household. The intent is not to make your home more like a factory, but rather to be open to changes that may make your life easier.

Worrying Is Work

Worrying has a negative reputation. We assume that worrying serves no purpose, that it consists of obsessing over worst-case scenarios and that it only leads to anxiety and wasted time. But we can consider worrying through another lens. Worrying can be considered cognitive labor and can sometimes be a worthy endeavor that brings value to your family. Let's consider: What does worrying entail?

Say you are going on a trip with your child who has a chronic medical condition. Worry may lead you down a path to imagine your child getting sick en route, or you've lost your luggage, or your needing to seek medical care while you're away. These worries can serve a purpose—and lead you to prepare for these scenarios. But the work of worrying takes time and energy and is often some of the most difficult work to outsource. No one cares enough about your child or knows enough about your child to worry like you can.

In addition to "worry work," there is planning work. You can sign your child up for a course of physical therapy and hire someone to take them to this weekly, but you still must remember when it starts, when it ends, when the next contract and payment are due, and which days the center is closed for holidays. You have to manage the relationship and communication with the physical therapist. You need to consider whether it's the right choice to use a physical therapy center, or whether there would be cheaper or more effective alternative ways to get your child the support they need. Without this time spent caring and planning, your child would not get the services they need. Even though this cognitive labor is often unseen and unpaid, it's still inherently valuable.

Family Imbalances in Caregiving

As we discuss building our caregiver skills, we have to address a particular elephant in the room: the balance of task allocation within a family unit. Optimizing one family member's ability to support their child in a challenge won't address the feelings of inequity, overwhelm, or resentment that can build up when one parent feels alone in the work of caregiving. Families come in all shapes and sizes, and each has their unique challenges in finding a balance of who does what. Single-parent families, whether by choice or due to other circumstances, sometimes have fewer family members with whom to share responsibilities. I will note, though, that many of the single-parent families I have worked with often come with engaged family supports—a grandparent, sibling, partner, or close friend (neighbor or "auntie")—who play a central role in sharing some parenting duties such as childcare, household management, or meal prep. In these families, the dynamic is not entirely as different as you might think from two-parent households, and skills for communicating and delegating tasks equitably remain useful. Gender identity and sexual orientation also impact how parents divide responsibilities. Some data suggest that homosexual two-parent households delegate tasks more equitably, but often one parent remains the default "breadwinner" and the other the "primary parent."[1]

If you follow the public dialogue led by writers Brigid Schulte, Jessica Grose, and Eve Rodsky, you'll probably have heard that the disparities in household labor within cisgender, heterosexual two-parent homes often tilt toward women, who carry a greater load of cognitive work. Sociologist Allison Daminger quantified this in her work profiling middle- and high-socioeconomic status two-parent households raising children under five in Boston, Massachusetts. Thirty-two of these couples were heterosexual cisgender couples, and when looking in detail, she found women did approximately 82 percent of the monitoring and 65 percent of the anticipating work.[2]

When household labor pertains to children and to health-related work, it's even more likely to be gender imbalanced. We know that in the US, mothers attend about 84 percent of visits to the pediatrician while fathers attend about 19 percent of visits.[3] A larger study from Israel concurs that when one parent attends a pediatric visit, it's the mother 76 percent of the time; and analysis in Denmark found that mothers handled 90 percent of health-care visits.[4] At the individual level, many factors may drive this trend, including which parent does more paid work and what parent preference is. Substantial cultural and societal norms may encourage mothers to be the main caregiver because of a perception that women are "better" at caregiving.[5] Pediatricians, myself included, may in some ways be part of the problem, reinforcing cultural norms by making assumptions about which parent to contact for health matters or by screening mothers for depression following childbirth without screening fathers.[6]

Perpetuating this default—that women handle the caregiving work and managing their family's interactions with health-care professionals—doesn't do anyone any good. We know that discrepancies in the sharing of household labor can increase resentment and marital conflict—variables that impact parent wellness and, inevitably, child outcomes. Additionally, when children have chronic health and educational needs, data (not surprisingly) suggest that when fathers are more involved, the child benefits—better child adherence to treatment, better child psychological adjustment, and improved health status.[7]

If you are struggling with allocating labor equitably in your home, some of the skills I'll discuss later in this chapter like communication and time management will help. But as a first step, I recommend improving awareness of who does what within your household. When you are open about what you are doing—especially if you are frustrated, overwhelmed, or sensing an imbalance—explicit, clear communication is the first step toward making a change. Sometimes more transparency inspires change directly—if your partner doesn't know how much is on your plate, they may not know when you need more help. Even if it doesn't motivate change, it can lead to acknowledgment and awareness as more work emerges to be done.[8]

While we can't immediately change the broader society or health and educational systems with which we interact, we can change the way our family works. Often time spent in this pursuit—allocating tasks more equitably or more thoughtfully—can have a large positive impact on family functioning. Before we dive into how to optimize your individual performance, consider:

- Do you communicate openly with your caregiving partners about all that you do?
- Do you feel resentment about the balance of tasks within your household?
- If you'd like to change the balance of caregiving responsibilities, what barriers have kept you from this in the past?

Skills to Help Optimize Your Performance

While it may feel odd to think of your parenting and caregiving "performance," objectively assessing how well you handle the work on your plate may help you to make meaningful improvements. As we discussed earlier, understanding your unique skills, strengths, and weaknesses can help you respond to your challenge in the best way. If you can have the cognitive flexibility to think of yourself objectively, as an employer might think about an employee, how would you review yourself? Some things are going well, and you have some areas for growth. Once you identify these areas, you can change and adapt for the better.

When you think of a job review, the domains offered for evaluation might include some of the following:

- Goal-setting and continuous improvement
- Time-management skills
- Communication skills
- Teamwork
- Organization
- Creativity
- Problem-solving

As you read this list, you probably picked out a few skills you know you already excel at. When you think about improving your performance, you can look at the area where you struggle and seek easy ways for meaningful improvement. If I give myself a low score in time management, making a small improvement might result in substantial found time. You might find different ways to improve your skills, perhaps by reading a book, setting some goals, or asking for help. It could also be helpful to really lean in to what you are best at—using your strengths to support your weaker areas. If you enjoy organization, can you take this skill and apply it to other areas, like communication or teamwork, to improve your performance?

There are a few reasons some parents may hesitate to set goals for their caregiving and home life. One of the most common barriers I encounter is pessimism or learned helplessness. Parents stop believing that things can be better. Hope and optimism are essential ingredients for setting goals. Goals can motivate creative problem-solving and enhanced performance. When someone makes a small positive change, they may see a small positive impact, which provides additional motivation and positive feedback to continue the process of change. But this starts with the bravery and self-confidence to consider that you can improve your family's experience of whatever you are facing.[9]

I believe you can make small meaningful changes and I hope you do too. However, as we proceed, let's keep in mind that your performance is often not the problem, though it may be part of the solution. The healthcare and educational systems you navigate are difficult. Our society doesn't prioritize and protect caregivers. But you have control over your behavior and choices. So, even if this doesn't fix the underlying problem, it may help.

Skill Building—An Incentive

Gloria immigrated from Mexico and only spoke Spanish. When I first started treating her children, I experienced some difficulty in our communication. I knew some Spanish, but her regional accent was thick, and her specific dialect used a lot of local colloquialisms that made it hard for me to comprehend. We used a telephone-based translation system, through which we connected with four translators from her region who could help, but when they weren't available, communication was difficult.

Even with adequate translation in place, Gloria was not familiar with the American health-care system. She wasn't sure how or when to access emergency services, and she had never worked with a pharmacy before, and her children's health suffered as a result. These barriers were not reflections on her intelligence, but gaps in her skill set and experience.

She knew she had to remedy the situation. She signed up for English language classes and frequently reached out to social workers for help accessing health care. Over time, she mastered English and gained medical fluency, and once her children were plugged in to care, Gloria used these skills to find paid work as a medical assistant.

Nothing about this was easy. Gloria hardly had the time, money, or childcare she needed to make this commitment. But she found a way, because she knew it was important to her family. The resilience caregiving parents exhibit is inspiring. While we think of our children as works in progress, sometimes we forget that adults can also change their habits, tendencies, and abilities.

Time Management

As a cancer survivor, despite being in good health, I have half a dozen health maintenance appointments a year. Keeping track of this requires a substantial amount of energy, particularly when circumstances in my life change—a new job schedule, a new health insurance carrier, or moving to a new address. Some of these specialists are in different hospital systems and don't communicate with each other. Some of the tests require prior authorization from insurance, and even when this is obtained there are at least a few bills per encounter. While I'd like to rely on my own primary care doctor to organize and execute this maintenance plan, in my early thirties I finally realized that ultimately, I cannot evade responsibility.

Accepting the scope of the responsibility was an important "aha" moment for me. I did the mental math with a certain number of appointments a year, each requiring a specific amount of time scheduling, traveling, and following up, and the final number was not one I was happy about. Only then, when I realized the total impact on my life and my family, how this work eroded time for the other things I wanted to do personally and professionally, did I commit to minimizing the unnecessary time.

This first step to creating a solid time-management plan is to understand what you are *already* doing and what you *need* to be doing. To accomplish this goal, you can start by tracking every task you complete during the day or how you spend every minute of your day. Many caregivers decrease their paid work to accommodate their caregiving responsibilities, but doing so does not mean their time becomes less valuable. Your time has value, so considering how you spend this valuable commodity is important.

Being selective and intentional about your time is an important part of improving your family life. At times you may need to compartmentalize some of your caregiving. Perhaps your other child needs your attention in a particular week, or you need to focus on your career, and you aren't able to devote the usual amount of time to caregiving. This may go against our instincts as parents, who often want everything for our children right away, but more often than not, you can put off some concerns and, in doing so, lighten your load.

As you look critically at how you spend your time, consider the following:

- What is the most important thing you do all week?
- Is there one thing you can just stop doing?
- If you had more time, what would you do with it?
- What are three ways you spend your time that bring you joy and you want to spend more time doing?

- What are the three things you do that you hate doing and wish you could eliminate?
- What are the factors (financial, practical, relational) that keep you from changing the way you spend your time? Are there any that could change?

Barriers to Intentionally Spending Your Time

When you take a critical look at how you are spending your time, you need to investigate what your priorities are. *Why* do you want to make these changes? What areas need more attention: your child's caregiving, the siblings or other family members, or your own well-being? When you break down how you are spending your time, you'll identify some items that you enjoy and value in your week, things that spark connections with loved ones or inspire your creativity. Before eliminating those tasks, ask yourself what it is you enjoy about them. Some self-awareness may help you identify more ways to increase joy.

You'll also find that you're using your time on things you didn't expect, such as spending more time than you realized on social media or watching TV. Some of this may be purpose-driven, or for relaxation or connection, but some of it may be filler. Some of us may find that we spend a lot of time doing things that we do not enjoy and that we are not particularly well suited for.

In her book *168 Hours*, Laura Vanderkam discusses options for clearing your calendar and recommends ignoring and minimizing these undesired tasks. Sometimes we find ourselves doing things, even time-consuming things, but when we think critically it doesn't have to be that way. Just letting a task go completely can be best. Early in the COVID-19 pandemic, my nurses were photographing and uploading each COVID-19 test from patients for record-keeping purposes. As we got busier and I took a closer look at our workflow, I realized we could stop documenting photos and simply write the result in the chart, saving time without sacrificing quality.

To minimize the time you spend, sometimes you can constrain time spent doing something into an allocated block—for example, set a limit for time spent scrolling social media or watching TV. Batching tasks can help reduce the time spent too. Rather than responding to each medical bill or insurance correspondence that comes in the mail immediately, allowing them to accumulate (within reason) and sitting down to handle several at once may be more efficient.

Other items that can't be minimized or omitted may be able to be delegated or outsourced to use less time. While many parents think of outsourcing as a luxury out of reach, remember that sometimes you can outsource or delegate *within* your family without an additional financial cost if you have a co-parent, a sibling, a grandparent, or a neighbor who may be willing. Some children with disabilities or dependence on medical technologies can qualify for home health aids, personal-care aids, or skilled nursing at home through their insurance or through Medicaid waiver programs. If you think your child might qualify for this type of assistance, ask your child's physician or a social worker for help.

However, even if you can outsource, you still must dedicate time to planning, coordination, and supervision. In addition to the financial barriers to outsourcing, sometimes relatively benign, well-intentioned thought processes interfere with making good decisions about which tasks we own versus which we delegate. If you can identify these cognitive errors, you can redirect your thoughts. For example:

- **"It's on me as the parent."** Some parents feel shame or stigma in asking for help, as if needing help indicates you are less capable or dedicated. To the contrary, I often feel impressed when I see a parent identify a possible need for their child and fill it.
- **"I do it better."** Often caregiving parents feel when their child is ill or suffering that there is no acceptable substitute for their presence. Sometimes this may be true, but often there are other loving adults willing to support your child. The largest barrier to delegating to these individuals is not their competence but your trust.

Sometimes parents truly are better, but for some less-essential tasks, it's also possible that someone else doing it imperfectly would be better than you doing it perfectly and suffering.

- **"It's easier for me to do it."** Especially when we are used to things being done a certain way, this is often true in the short-term. But for tasks that will require a long-term commitment, you do stand to accrue a long-term benefit by investing the time required to train someone else and delegate. Imagine cleaning up after dinner or packing a bag for school; it may take months or years to teach your children to do these tasks reliably, but once they do, they have gained a skill and you have gained daily assistance.

As you consider the structure of your workday as a caregiver, one of the most obvious ways in which a parent differs from a paid employee is break time and leave. Few parents protect their need for a break—a meal, a shower, or chat with a friend. You can't ever truly be off duty as a parent in the same way as with paid work. But we know that vacation, rest, and leisure make employees more effective, and you deserve these benefits too.

Later in Chapter 7, we'll talk more about how we balance care between co-parents and delegate some of these tasks to your co-caregiver or other people in your life. While there are many barriers to successfully assigning these tasks to others, frequently it becomes a necessity.

Communication: Teach-Back

As we've discussed, most children have a team of people involved in their care—teachers during and after school, therapists, babysitters, and family who aren't always involved day to day. Even when children aren't facing challenges, keeping everyone informed can be a time-consuming task—what does your child want to eat, what's the routine for sleep, what do they wear are all essential pieces of information constantly changing.

When a child is facing a challenge, the quantity of information and the essential nature of the information multiplies—medications, therapies, appointments, doctors' phone numbers, emergency plans, and supplies. If there were a time when you could fully train everyone and just be done with it, that would be one thing, but a child is always changing and so is their plan.

Informing family of a plan to give medication or to pick a child up from a certain address a certain day can be seem straightforward, but many challenges involve care plans that can bring up individual opinions, values, and beliefs. Diet, discipline, use of medication, making a big deal out of something, or maintaining vigilance about a safety plan are the type of issues I see frequently cause drama between parents and other members of the care team. Fear of judgment and stigma can become barriers to communication. Communication about other conditions such as mental health, disabilities, or genetic conditions can similarly be more complicated to discuss openly, especially with many stakeholders.

As a caregiving parent, you'll find that you know more about your child than anyone else does, sometimes even more than your medical or educational team does. But there will be times when others are caring for, teaching, coaching, or supervising your children. To effectively quarterback your child's care, you have to share your knowledge with others productively and keep them updated over time. An essential part of this is to build in time and opportunity for communication. When you leave a meeting with a teacher at the school or a physician in a clinic, it's a good practice to consider not just what you need to do, but who you need to inform about the conversation. You can also consider regular meeting times to solicit feedback from other caregivers on how things are going. When you listen to these other important people in your child's life, you can learn important information to improve your child's care plan. You can also share important updates and priorities for their time with your child.

It's essential for parents to be thoughtful about minimizing errors and maximizing understanding. The Agency for Healthcare Research and Quality (AHRQ) has developed a "Health Literacy Universal Precautions Toolkit," which is designed to help medical providers communicate more effectively with patients. Their data show that only 12 percent of individuals receiving instructions from their provider understand them. The education level of the individual is only one of many barriers here; often, health professionals use jargon and convey complex topics quickly—particularly when emotions are high, or an individual is not feeling well or focused. Similarly, when you communicate between a caregiving parent and another family member or paid caregiver, there may be a misunderstanding.

To tackle this problem, one of the tools the AHRQ promotes is called "teach-back." Teach-back was designed for health-care providers to use with their patients, but this tool can be used by caregiving parents when they are communicating their child's care plan with others. You are now the expert in your child and you are instructing others, so using similar techniques makes sense. Teach-back involves asking the receiver of information to explain what they've just been told. The goal isn't to test their verbatim recall; if they repeat your words back to you, that doesn't mean what you said was understood. The goal is to see how they have interpreted what you've said.

Say a parent brings their child into the emergency room after their child has had a seizure. After a workup, my team concludes it is a febrile seizure and I explain what that means.[10] Next, I'd say, "I have just given you a lot of information about your child's febrile seizures. It's important for you to understand, and I know you've been through a lot today. Because this is important, I want you to pretend that I'm a friend or family member who you'll be sharing this information with, so I can be certain what I've told you is clear and accurate."

Though many parents are shy to begin this exercise, once they do, I can congratulate them and validate what they do understand well and correct whatever they misunderstand. Even the most conscientious, educated parent misses things sometimes, either because I was unclear, their attention wandered, or they were tripped up by jargon.

You can also practice this at home. If you're just starting out with a new diagnosis, you might say to your co-parent, teacher, or babysitter, "I've been learning so much about this new challenge, and I can't recall exactly how much I've shared. Would you mind just summarizing your understanding of what my child's diagnosis and plan are, so I can be certain we're on the same page?"

This big check-in might feel overwhelming, especially at first, so you can start slowly or with a more specific topic. "I really want to ensure we don't make a mistake with this medicine, so can you show me how you'll pull up the dose?" While it can feel awkward at first, incorporating teach-back is a very effective tool for making sure your child is getting the best care.

Teach-back can also help with assessing the big picture understanding of those on your team. In my work with children with type 1 diabetes, I frequently encountered families with personal experience with type 2 diabetes. This may appear to be an advantage—a family member with diabetes might be more adept at monitoring blood sugars, identifying the symptoms of high blood sugar, and understanding why it's important to control the sugars. Unfortunately, this is not always the case.

Type 2 diabetes responds to lifestyle modifications in a way that type 1 diabetes does not. An individual with type 2 diabetes is less sensitive to the effects of insulin and has some ability to control elevated blood sugar by changing behavior—exercise, diet, sleep, and maintaining a healthy weight. That said, medication is often an important component of care for people with type 2 diabetes. Type 1 diabetes is actually an autoimmune disease wherein the body has attacked the pancreas; the pancreas is essentially burnt-out and produces no insulin. This means that, for these kids, life with diabetes will be different—their blood sugars will never be normal without insulin; they will always be fully dependent on insulin.

But, if you have a family member, nurse, or babysitter who has experience managing type 2 diabetes, they might not fully understand that the child's blood sugar spikes are not due to their behaviors or dietary habits. They may be inclined to blame the child, which is fundamentally unfair. The goal should be to help these children live and enjoy their best lives, while providing the insulin they need.

If these parents use teach-back to communicate with their caregivers to assess their understanding, they can be sure that the caregivers truly understand the condition so they can provide the best care. If the people involved in your child's life don't understand the foundations of your child's condition, they may make errors or mismanage your child's care. To refer back to the example above, the "why" of the high blood sugar makes all the difference in how you form your plan and the tone of your day-to-day communications with the child. Checking for understanding of the details and the big picture is an important piece of your work.

An Organized Approach

The next piece of optimizing your performance centers on how you are structuring your work. It's not unusual for caregiving work to come unexpectedly and begin with a period of uncertainty. For example, James was a twelve-year-old boy in the care of his grandmother. He looked pale and seemed to be growing more slowly than his peers, so she brought him to the pediatrician. When his blood counts were found to be just one-third of the normal level, he was urgently admitted to the hospital. Testing showed that, despite having no abdominal pain and a good appetite, he had blood in his stool and wasn't absorbing nutrients well. A gastroenterologist performed an endoscopy, which confirmed a diagnosis of inflammatory bowel disease. His grandmother left the hospital with new prescriptions, follow-up appointments with several providers, and a discharge summary in a big folder.

A few years later, James was thriving with his diagnosis and showed up for an intake with me as his new pediatrician. Grandmother handed over the same overflowing, taped-together folder with documentation from more than twenty appointments, insurance paperwork about medication approvals, some camp and school forms, and partial records of dozens of different prescriptions. The folder had all the essential information and some organization. While it was not navigable for me, the packet was working for her. During our discussion, when she would need to reference a detail, she could find what she needed after digging around for a few moments. But when she got up to leave, she dropped the folder, and hundreds of papers mixed up in a big pile on the floor. She almost cried—curating his records took time she didn't have. While the folder strategy was not doing harm, it certainly was not helping.

My social worker and a hospital volunteer were able to help her. I printed out a one-page summary of James's medications and current doctors with upcoming appointments, and we added a few other key records—a growth chart and vaccine summary. My social worker and the volunteer found a hole-puncher and an extra three-ring binder and organized his records—not perfectly, but enough so that a few duplicates could be tossed and the important records wouldn't go missing. We hoped this new model would help the grandmother in the process of following up with multiple specialists, dealing with school accommodations, and insurance battles of medication, but she was mostly excited to leave the three-ring binder at home and not carry the whole pile to every visit.

Investing effort in an organizational plan will help maximize your efficiency and save you time in the long-term. Only you can know what works best for your family and the systems you interact with, but all caregiving parents should be sure to organize their medical information, their space, and their caregiving work. So, let's break down all three.

Organizing Your Medical Information

Caregiving parents should create or be given by their doctors a care plan. This is an invaluable tool and contains a list of essential contacts for your child's care (doctors, therapists, educators, etc.), a list of medications and equipment, a list of upcoming appointments, and a running list of questions or concerns.

Example of a Care Plan

Name: Anna
Care Plan Date: 10/9/2022
Date of Birth: 6/15/2016
Medical Record Number: 7233947
Allergies: Walnuts, Amoxicillin
Last Weight: 56 lb
Medical summary / List diagnoses:
Anna was born at 32 weeks premature. She has asthma, reflux, and food and drug allergies. She is nearsighted and wears glasses. She has mild cerebral palsy, wears ankle foot orthotic braces, and received physical therapy.

Care Team

	Contact info	Date of Last Visit	Next appt.	Notes
Dr. Fradin (Pediatrician)	555-555-5555	12/5/2021	3/5/2022	
Eye Doctor	555-555-5555	1/15/2022	1/2023	In local office Tuesdays and Fridays
Dentist	555-555-5555	8/1/2021	4/10/2022	
Dr. Allergist	555-555-5555	12/2021	12/2022	
Dr. Rehabilitation	555-555-5555	6/2021	12/2022	
PT	555-555-5555	Tuesdays	Ends 5/21/2022	Next IEP 3/2022

Medication List

Lansoprazole Medication for reflux	10 ml once a day	Filled at pharmacy A 777-777-7777	Call a week before refill for prior authorization on Wednesday between 12:00 p.m. and 5:00 p.m.
Montelukast Medication for asthma	Chewable tablet at bedtime	Filled at pharmacy A	
Epinephrine Medication for food allergy	Use only if needed	Filled at pharmacy B 777-7777-7777	
Ankle foot orthotics	New order can be placed on 2/2022	Supply store C 888-888-8888	Will need an appointment to measure and reorder with Dr. Rehabilitation.

This is a concise tool that parents can share with caregivers from baby-sitters to teachers, and parents can bring this tool to appointments with doctors and therapists to ensure everyone is up-to-date. Parents should be sure to date the care plan so that if the specific details have been changed, you can know whether someone has the most up-to-date version.

Some families prefer a tangible resource like a notebook or use an annual planner to organize their child's care—finding it easier to jot notes as things come up. Other families use a digital resource like a shared document in a cloud—this can allow information updated to the minute, and everyone with access to the document will have access to the most updated version. There are other useful electronic tools families can use to organize their care. Electronic calendar notifications can remind you when refills will be due or when authorizations need to be renewed, or to set reminders about future follow-ups before you leave the doctor's office.

Keeping a file or a few files with reference information about your child's medical condition can also be helpful. Most of the time you may not need the original reports from when they were diagnosed, but you never know when something might again be relevant if you move or initiate care with a new provider. Digitizing these files and giving them specific file names with dates can make them even easier to find. Similarly, having a saved and searchable list of contacts and resources can be essential so you don't end up doing the excess work of finding information again and again.

I recommend that all families keep a list of emergency contacts and medications posted in a central part of the home, such as taped to the inside of a kitchen cabinet. This simple safety step is even more important if you have a child with a special health need in your home.

Organizing Your Space

Many families acquire a lot of supplies and medical equipment and need to consider the best ways to organize and store them. We want to keep medication out of reach of young children, yet accessible for parents. Ideally medication should be kept in a cool, dark space; sunlight, heat, and humidity extremes (like shower steam!) can degrade the potency of the medication over time.

Some families store medications for too long, instead of checking expiration dates regularly and throwing out expired medication. Some families actually have a hard time letting go of the leg braces that have been outgrown or will hold on to excess medication and formula just in case. Retaining supplies that are expired or no longer functional can take up important space, and the clutter can make it harder for you to find the medications you need when you need them. I recommend periodically seeing what equipment you can pass along or what medications you can discard.[11]

Parents often find the process of getting young children out of the house to be cumbersome and time-consuming, especially during that time crunch before work or school. When you add in medications, safety devices, glasses, and the extra equipment or extra time required for some children, the process can become even more chaotic. Families can ease the process—and avoid doubling back for forgotten items—by using a checklist as part of the routine before leaving the house. Other families may find bedtime to be the difficult time of day. Structuring your space thoughtfully to make sure you have what you need at the pain points of your day can make things more manageable.

Organizing Your Caregiving Work

Many families don't anticipate a lot of work at home. You might get a bill and pay it, but often there isn't a workplace-style routine established for efficiently tackling complex projects in the home.

When you are parenting a child through a challenge, however, you will find yourself managing complex projects at home. Take a moment to consider if you have allocated space in your home where you can sit down and handle the typical inevitable errands that come up. In this space there should be pens, pencils, Post-its, envelopes, stamps, a checkbook, a copy of your care plan and insurance card, and all the contact information you might need. If you don't have a set place where you tackle tasks like this, you may find yourself spending extra time finding these key supplies every time an errand comes up.

You may find that batching tasks improves your efficiency. Instead of dealing with tasks as they come in, you can set aside a time to sit down and charge through many of them at once. Many of these tasks are routine and can be batched fairly easily, like the medication refills, the medical bills, or the school's requests for paperwork. The benefit of batching this work is that not only do you get the work done potentially more efficiently, but you also make that work less of a nuisance during the other times of your week when the interruption might derail you from all of the other things you do. We are notoriously worse at multitasking than we think we are. Trying to find some time in your day to single-task can promote creativity and improve your performance. Maintaining an organizational system can prevent last-minute emergencies and decrease stress.

In this chapter, we've discussed a lot of logistics for how your family tackles the complexity of parenting a child through a challenge. This chapter may leave you feeling like there are a lot of opportunities to improve things—whether it's the way you allocate labor with your co-parent, spend your time, communicate with your team, or organize your life. Please remember that perfection is not the goal. Sometimes one small change can be a big help—decreasing your stress, increasing your ability to focus, or freeing up a tiny bit more of your time to relax or play.

In the next chapter we're going to talk more about promoting healthy dynamics with others in your home—your co-parents, extended family members, friends, and your child's siblings. Before we move on consider:

- Is there one area—delegating tasks, time management, communi-
  cating, or organizing—where you feel you'd like to improve?
- What would be the benefit of making changes?
- What barriers have kept you from doing this in the past?
- Are there resources that would help you improve the way you're
  managing all these logistics?

CHAPTER 7

Taking Inventory of the Rest of Your Family

In my complex-care practice, I often had residents who were training to be pediatricians spend time with me to learn more about helping families facing challenges. For a few weeks, I worked with Elana, a very eager third-year resident hoping to find a job in a similar practice. Ahead of her first visit with a patient, I made sure she knew the history and goals of the visit, and she went in to talk to the family and examine the child.

A few minutes later, she returned and presented me with a summary of the child's case. Elana started with why the child had been brought in for a visit that day, detailed her exam, and shared a tentative plan. Elana was thorough, she had done a truly excellent job, but I interrupted her before she could further discuss her assessment and plan.

"Who brought the patient?" I asked. Her eyes went blank—she hadn't asked. A new doctor always remembers to introduce himself or herself, but often makes assumptions about who is present at the visit. Anyone can bring a patient to a visit—it could be a parent, a sibling, a nurse, a grandparent, or an "auntie" or "uncle" (who often is not at all related to the patient). But not everyone is equally knowledgeable and reliable regarding the child's status. The source of information is essential to understanding the story and making an appropriate diagnosis and plan. When we discovered it was a new nurse who had brought the child in, Elana called the patient's mom. With a better understanding of why the child needed our help, we were able to make a better plan.

Just as I need to understand who is involved and see things from their perspective, you need to be aware of your own family ecosystem. Your family members are some of your most valued assets—they can help you and support you and love you, but they also have their own limitations and needs that require attention. When you grow up within this eco-system, you *know* what you can and can't ask of your family members. You know who to turn to when you are looking for specific kinds of sup-port and who to avoid with certain hot-button issues. If you make these dynamics more explicit, you may see things more clearly, including the potential for change.

Consider Alex, a child with sensory processing issues. Being around him takes patience. He won't wear weather-appropriate clothes, loud noises cause him to melt down, and his restrictive diet has warranted professional involvement from nutritionists, feeding therapists, and a gastroenterologist. Perhaps his mother was raised in an authoritarian, "clean your plate" household and, as a result, is reluctant to discuss the issue with her own mother—the first few times the mother mentioned his health issues, Grandma suggested she just needed to be more firm.

If you have a family member or caregiver on your team who you think of as judgmental or uninformed, you may stop keeping them in the loop. It may feel like too much of a drain on your energy, adding stress to an already challenging parenting situation. One choice is to tell them less about the day-to-day situation and not share how things are progressing or the insights of specialist visits. You may choose to do this for a good reason, for example to reserve your energy for other priorities, but in doing so you will decrease the chances the situation will improve. Your caregiver will be even less capable of learning, catching up, and adjusting their attitude to one that is more productive. The gap between where you are and where they are will widen over time.

Your options are to "give up" on finding a way to integrate them into your family life or to try and find a way to help them get to where they need to be to support your journey. You can provide context and education, set expectations, and follow through with boundaries to make their engagement in your child's life safer and more pleasant for all. This work will take energy, but expecting them to learn and change without your guidance and involvement may be unrealistic. To that end, in this chapter we'll discuss some strategies for getting family members on board when one or more of your children is facing challenges.

Families come in all shapes and sizes. Many parents are single parents. While some of the language of this section may invoke the idea of a traditional nuclear family, including a spouse, with many of the families I work with, the co-parent is effectively an aunt, grandmother, or babysitter. Whatever type of parenting partner(s) you have, you need a plan for how you share the efforts of meeting your challenge.

As a parent, you have a lifelong commitment to your child and love them unconditionally, but you do not have to be a parent to partner in parenting or caregiving. So many families have grandparents, aunts and uncles, cousins, or close friends who are part of their day in and day out life. Anyone who is truly invested in your child, who loves them and who you can count on to consistently help, can for the purposes of this discussion be considered a co-parent.

In many situations, hired help, including babysitters, teachers, or nurses, fall into a different category. I have seen magic happen when these professionals become integrated and develop a relationship based on something deeper than a contract or a salary. If you are lucky enough to have a helper who becomes someone you can really depend on, protect and support that relationship.

Why You Need a Co-caregiver

Arturo was a teenager with tuberous sclerosis, a genetic condition that predisposes to developmental delay, intellectual disability, tumor formation, and epilepsy. He was unable to communicate verbally and had behavioral issues that precluded his participation in school. He and his mother were very close, and no one knew how to manage his behavior but her. Her family mostly lived elsewhere, and his father was not involved. She knew the early warning signals that indicated an imminent meltdown, and she knew how to reroute her son to avoid them. She was the one facilitating home school, feeding him every meal, helping with his daily needs, and getting him to sleep each night.

I saw that she was doing all this work on her own, without a break, and I worried for her well-being. Every time I saw her and Arturo, I asked about respite. When does she get a break to see her friends or visit her family? Who helps her and how can we get her more help? Mostly she would push off my concerns, and I would respectfully back off. But one year, she said she was glad I asked. Her mother was ill, and she needed to travel to go and see her. We'd need to find a place for Arturo to stay for two weeks in about three to six months. We rallied the social work team and arranged for Arturo's mom to visit the options covered by his insurance. Around that time, disaster struck.

Arturo's mom contracted an infection of her gallbladder and gallstones, and she was hospitalized and required emergency surgery. It was now urgent that we find extra help for Arturo. Luckily, since we had a head start on some of the approvals and paperwork, we were able to get Arturo placed within a few days in a subacute nursing facility where children with special health-care needs sometimes stayed to recover from surgery or to provide their families with respite. Unfortunately, while waiting for the insurance approval and bed allocation process, Arturo had to be held in the pediatric emergency room and hospital unit for two days to facilitate the transition, an uncomfortable and inconvenient situation.

Arturo was worried about his mother, but he managed fairly well in the subacute nursing facility. His mom saw that others were capable of stepping up to care for him—not as well as she did, but well enough to ensure his safety and comfort. He returned to the facility at least annually thereafter, whenever his mom was unable to care for him for an extended period of time—due to health or personal reasons.

Arturo's mom was devoted to him, but part of being an effective caregiver is recognizing that you can't *always* be there. It's not always best for the child when one caregiver is managing a situation alone. While one person may own a given part of caregiving, such as administering the medications, another caregiver needs to be prepared to step in if needed. When a parent includes others in caregiving, this will also increase the quality of the care. While sometimes we shy away from sharing work because others approach things differently, there is also the opportunity for improvement when we gain a new perspective.

When a parent has a partner in caregiving, another important upside is the possibility of finding more joy and connection with others. In my work, I've had jobs where I had a robust team, as well as a solo practice where I was relatively alone in my work. Working alone, I missed having an opportunity to celebrate the wins with others, as well as the chance to vent frustrations. Similarly, when one caregiver is managing a situation alone, it can lead to isolation, frustration, and burnout. When these issues are left unaddressed long-term, this can lead to depression.

If you have been doing all of the caregiving work alone, I urge you to find partners in this work. Sometimes I speak with single parents without local family members, who are in situations with few obvious supports, as with Arturo's mom. Financial and practical limitations to finding caregiving support are difficult barriers. Sometimes parents can find meaningful connections and support from neighbors, religious institutions, or other parents of children with special health-care needs. I've also found that even parents with engaged and loving co-parents still feel alone in the work of caregiving. We have to be realistic and open-minded about who the best candidates are who might be able to help you, and for many families we have to think outside of the traditional box of your co-parent being the only person able to functionally engage in this caregiving work.

What are the root causes that lead us to remain alone in our caregiving responsibilities? As you'll see in the examples below, often difficult feelings underly our hesitation with practical consequences:

- **Guilt:** AJ had been born prematurely with developmental impairments and had a long stay in the NICU. AJ's mom seemed to be furious all the time. It took me a few months to realize that she was mostly angry at herself. She blamed herself for his preterm birth, and she punished herself by pushing away support. His premature birth was not her fault, and even if it were somehow, she still was worthy of support, and her son was still deserving of the best care. AJ's mom had unresolved feelings of guilt that led her to behave like a martyr.

- **Shame:** Neveah's mom was tough. She had overcome a lot of adversity and worked really hard to not need help from others. She did not want pity and she certainly didn't want any help. Whenever Neveah's health took a bad turn and Neveah's mom needed support, we would review the list of people in her life. She didn't want the neighbors, her boss, or her uncle to know what she was facing. Some of what kept her from opening up to these individuals were her feelings of shame. She was understandably proud of where she was and what her daughter had accomplished, and she worried that others would diminish those feelings and see her family in a more vulnerable and negative light.

- **A need for control:** Laura's mother had considered her options and decided none were good enough. Her child's grandmother made too many snide comments, her husband worked too much, and her sister had questionable judgment. But underlying her struggle was her need for perfection and control. For Laura, the anxiety that she felt coping with her child's challenge had only been soothed when she was doing everything herself in a way that was up to her standards.

I can't know you and your family personally, but frequently in addition to the financial and logistic barriers to getting help, emotions stand in the way. I'd encourage you to dig deeper and consider whether your guilt, shame, or anxiety might be keeping you from getting the help you'd like in supporting your child. In the next section, I'll tackle some strategies for collaborating with a co-caregiver.

Successfully Collaborating with a Co-caregiver

One family I worked with had an organized and successful mother who knew every detail of her daughter's medical care. Her daughter had been born premature at just twenty-four weeks, and her main medical issue was chronic lung disease due to prematurity. She needed oxygen and had a tracheostomy—a breathing tube—in her neck that we hoped she'd outgrow as she became bigger and stronger. Her mother's brain held every action item relating to her daughter's health, the inventory of supplies and medications at home, the name of every nurse they used at night and every doctor they had seen, as well as when a refill or follow-up visit would be necessary. She didn't just know her daughter's history; she knew all the past dates of procedures and symptoms, when dosages had been adjusted, and she deeply understood the pathology of her daughter's underlying condition.

But it was the dad who was with the daughter most during the day. He knew a bit more about the daughter's personality, her tastes, preferences, and her activities. When he showed up for visits, he was never shy about his limitations. He did not necessarily know the medications or the details, and in most visits would immediately get the "decision-maker" mom on the phone.

But Dad's perspective was valuable and important. When I would coax his participation, he would chime in with specific observations about what he saw, adding comments like, "Last night was bad, but I don't think she's coughed once today." He had a strong intuition about his daughter's wellness and when something seemed wrong, he didn't always know why but he always knew to say something and collaborate to figure it out.

What I loved about their balance was the mutual respect—at times he would say things like, "I am the one who is doing the day-to-day caring and she is the one driving the bus." Their arrangement was not entirely equitable, as he was devoting more hours to childcare, but they both had a sense of peace about the situation and could talk about it without tension.

Finding balance between two parents can be a challenge—your workload and the complexity of what you manage day-to-day increases substantially when you have children. When you have caregiving responsibilities on top of this, you are navigating not just co-parenting but also co-caregiving. If it's rare for parenting responsibilities to be equitably and fairly divided, it's even more unusual to have caregiving responsibilities that are easily divisible. Someone is always at more appointments, doing more research, or present at more therapy sessions. There's nothing wrong with this—it simply reflects the reality of most households. Depending on work outside the home and childcare responsibilities, every family has to find their unique balance, and things can shift as needs change over time.

What's nonnegotiable is that all members of the caregiving team need to feel their contributions are valued and that all are in the loop enough to be part of important conversations. As you think about where you are and where you are going, it's helpful to have goals. When I imagine the ideal co-caregiving dynamic, I look for the following:

- Appreciation, shared understanding, and mutual respect
- Fairness and equity
- Clear boundaries, with flexibility

One of the most common problems is having work go unseen. Often primary caregivers do dozens or even hundreds of tasks that their partner or family do not know about. Only when your work is known can it feel appreciated. You can't have flexibility when one caregiver doesn't know what the other is doing. To stay connected, especially if you are starting out on the caregiving journey or a new facet of it, caregiving partners should share both the roses and the thorns. Partners should regularly discuss the best and worst parts of their day and listen deeply to each other. While you may crave a break from thinking about your caregiving duties at the end of the day, it's important to share basic insights with your partner about how you are spending your time.

If one caregiver feels overburdened or marginalized, resentment can grow. "You aren't helping," can become, "You don't care." Resentment can lead to hostility and damage the quality of the relationship. Children pick up on this tension and it can sometimes affect them—they may have trouble sleeping or experience behavioral setbacks due to this stress. If you're already in this situation, you know it can be self-perpetuating. Anger and resentment can impair communication and lead to more frustration. But it doesn't have to continue in this way.

With any relationship, there is give and take, and there may be times when your balance goes well and times when it's a disaster. But you can reset the balance and establish a new status quo. We all only have so much time and energy, so as you make a plan to divide and conquer, consider what you need. It helps to consider all the strengths and weaknesses of your caregiving team.

If one person is staying home and one is at the office, there are still ways to outsource tasks to the working spouse, such as insurance paperwork, scheduling appointments, or research. One parent may be more extroverted and enjoy the process of interviewing babysitters or informational interviewing parents who have been in your shoes. The more introverted parent may prefer tasks that can be done online or independently. If both caregivers are working outside the home, and paid caregivers are helping at home, you may want to invest time in their training to maximize their competencies.

A clear delineation of your responsibilities will set you up for success. If you have been at this for a while and are already feeling burnt-out or resentful, set the stage for a discussion by finding a time to talk. Do not let these concerns come out late at night unexpectedly or wait until you have reached your limit to vent frustrations. If you want the conversation to be productive, you need to speak up when you are both calm and have the energy to communicate well. When you talk, use "I" statements, such as "I'm overwhelmed," or, "I'm unhappy that I do not have enough time for ____." Have some specific and realistic ideas for change, and remain open to your partner's suggestions. Try to assume the good intent in your co-caregiver even if he or she has not been there for you in the ways you have wanted. Physical affection can help to heal feelings of resentment.

The happiest parents I have worked with had a plan for division of labor and didn't hesitate to share it. I once asked a caregiver about a patient's home nursing care, and before I could finish the question, they said, "Oh, we've got to get my partner on the phone; he manages this." Even if a division of labor is unequal, having a clear plan implies a mutual understanding and visibility for all labor.

Other times, I've met with caregivers who were less forthright about the caregiving dynamic between caregiving partners, and as a result, I misunderstood who was managing what in the household. If you are not normally the one to take the child to a visit, or not the parent concerned with the child's day-to-day care, it's better to tell the doctor what you don't know rather than make a best guess to make it seem like you know more than you do. If you don't speak up about what you don't know, this hampers my ability to understand your child's condition and may lead to misdiagnosis, an unrealistic plan, or the wrong prescription or refer-ral. Just as you benefit from knowing who does what, your care team benefits from an understanding of who is an expert at what part of the caregiving and what's happening in your day-to-day life.

Your Outer Circle

One of my patients, Neal, was having a really hard time with severe ulcerative colitis. At only twelve, his colon had become so inflamed that he had a lot of pain and malnutrition, but this was not even his chief concern. His case was so difficult, he required placement of an ostomy. Surgeons had redirected his colon, so instead of having a bowel movement the typical way into the toilet, his bowels emptied to a bag attached to his abdomen.

As you can imagine for a tween, having a bag of poop attached to you can be difficult on many levels. Practically, it affects how you move, and affects your comfort and clothing. You worry about your looks and smell even more than most children your age. And you may need more help than you want to have, which is particularly difficult for an adolescent who wants to explore their independence.

This is why I encouraged Neal's mother to bring in more family members for training. She had a job and other children—inevitably I thought someone may need to know how to use an ostomy bag other than Neal and his mother.

For this family, as for many others, when I urged them to broaden their support network, I got the hard stop. There was no one else the mom and child trusted with this sort of thing. As the family broke it down, I learned that the dad was too squeamish, the grandmother made rude comments, and the older brother made the child feel embarrassed. "It's just me," the mother insisted.

Each family draws the lines differently. There are true partners in caregiving—your inner circle—and then there are others who are part of your household's everyday life. Your outer circle may include people not genetically related to you—good friends, neighbors, business partners, babysitters, and anyone who is part of your daily life.

For this family, we ended up deciding that the school nurse was willing and able to serve as an extra resource. Since she was physically present at times when Mom wasn't, we could make a plan for her to take the ostomy care to the next level and add more support to the family, though it wasn't easy. The nurse's office wasn't private enough and the single-stall bathrooms weren't large enough, so we ended up asking the principal for help finding an appropriate place.

Our relationships with our outer circle can be complicated, and amidst a challenge, even more so. This family was not unique in identifying obstacles to gaining support from other family members. Practical issues like schedule and consistent availability can preclude involvement. Emotional barriers can come up, like insensitivity or lack of acceptance.

As the primary caregiver, you may also face difficulties bringing family members on board. You may struggle with worries like the following:

- Talking to your family about your child's challenge may trigger difficult feelings, making the problem seem bigger or more real.
- You don't think they can "get it" or contribute in a positive way.
- You worry that new stressors will bring out old patterns of dysfunction.

However, for many people, family is a free source of unconditional support. Our goal is to take as much of the good as we can and harness useful resources for the benefit of the caregiver and child. We have to understand the reality that family members have to learn to accept the challenge and learn about the child's condition to be helpful. We can appreciate that family members have strengths and weaknesses and limitations. Someone may be very loving but not reliable, or someone may be very willing to help but have to be told specifically what to do.

As you navigate building your family up to be as helpful as they can be, it's easy to put training and communicating with your extended circle as your last priority. You may have a list of ten direct and tangible things that you have to do today. But this goes back to identifying nonurgent, important priorities. If it's important for you and your child to count on these outside supports, you need to invest the time and energy in getting them involved in a way that can be productive. Even intrinsically "good" grandparents, neighbors, and best friends often have no idea what parents face or how they can fit in to be helpful. To harness these resources:

- **Give updates before waiting for certainty.** So often, parents defer speaking to loved ones until they have a diagnosis or a plan because they do not want to worry their loved ones. But often these family members know something is off and without details they assume the worst. Since it will take time to get folks up to speed, involving them in the process early, even by a short text, will help them to be there when you may need their help.
- **Set boundaries that are clear and consistent.** If your child is struggling with school, stating expectations will help your family members avoid worsening the situation. You may want to say, "Academics have been a challenge recently, and we're working on developing a plan. Please don't give him a hard time about his grades." Do not be surprised when these boundaries are violated, but do speak up, as at least some of these mistakes may be unintentional due to misunderstanding or habit.
- **Don't hesitate to ask for help with getting your family up to speed.** Your doctor, nurse, therapist, or school administrator can either speak with them directly or offer resources. If you have a lot on your plate, training extended family members may be something you can delegate.

Sometimes, even when you do everything right, you may hit a wall. We all have loved ones with true limitations. As much as you want and need them to get up to speed, they may not be able to. If you hit this point, you may feel angry and disappointed, and you may grieve. Even when we are parents ourselves, if a parent (like your child's grandparent) doesn't live up to expectations, it can be very disorienting. Seeing the limitation for what it is can also help save your energy from hoping or waiting for support that's not going to happen.

Siblings Are More Than Little Helpers

A child in crisis can throw off the family dynamic, and one of the most urgent priorities is to balance the needs of the other children in the home. Siblings, whether they are facing their own challenges or are in good health, are an important part of your family life. It's important to maintain your connection and presence in their life, and to facilitate their relationship with their siblings. So, how do you do this, and what obstacles can you anticipate in this process?

Being a sibling of a child facing a challenge can be incredibly stressful; frequently, they experience all of the worries and emotions a parent does, but they may have less capacity to cope. Evidence, while limited, suggests that we are right to be concerned for their well-being. Having a sibling with chronic illness may increase one's risk of anxiety and depression, decrease engagement with peer activities, and harm cognitive development scores.[1] These effects are significant statistically, but that doesn't mean these experiences are universal, inevitable, or large enough to make a meaningful difference in these children's lives. Despite the weight of watching a sibling struggle, many siblings thrive.

One of my most remarkable patients had just such a sibling. I cared for a set of eight-year-old twins born extremely premature with many medical complications—cerebral palsy, vision and hearing difficulties, and learning disabilities. One of the twins was more medically fragile and was hospitalized often for breathing difficulties. Though I saw the twins almost monthly and knew their mom well, I only saw their teenage brother a handful of times.

Each time, his maturity and insight into their experiences blew me away. His family members were recent immigrants without other family nearby. Like many in the Bronx, they lived with significant financial strain. Even so, he was number one in his class and attended a prestigious college on a full scholarship. I couldn't help but ask his mom, who was a single parent, how she did it.

She corrected me. "He did it," she insisted, her eyes shining with pride. He was a hardworking, loving, and emotionally strong young man. But when I pushed, it was clear that she had also thoughtfully prioritized his needs even when things got tough.

Sometimes that meant leaving her sick child in the hospital alone one evening so that she could have a meal with the older brother. While it was difficult to compartmentalize this way, this mother managed to have a conversation about her healthy child's middle school sports and science fair project when all she could think of was whether her sick child was showing signs of improvement in the hospital or heading toward admission in the ICU. Of course, there were times when physically being present for him wasn't possible, but the effort she invested helped her remain connected to him and have insight into his experience.

In addition, despite not having family nearby, she had sought out a small community and made sure he always had someone to talk to even if, at times, that meant requiring him to see a counselor at school. As he matured, she invited his input on decisions that affected the entire family and encouraged him to do things important to him even if it wasn't easy—like a summer internship in his area of interest or going away to school despite that she would have less help with the younger children.

Without knowing it, this mother had provided her son with exactly the kind of unconditional support evidence shows helps children overcome stress. From one perspective, having a struggling sibling can be traumatic, inciting fear and uncertainty into a child's life and requiring them to be more independent at a younger age. From another perspective, the experience promotes the development of skills and coping strategies. When supported appropriately, seeing firsthand that an adverse experience can be approached and survived can inspire resilience and develop character. While all parents try to teach inclusion, when a healthy child sees the world through the perspective of a child facing a challenge, they learn empathy and see their values in action. In the conversations I had with siblings while researching this book, I learned that many use friends' reactions to their sick sibling as a barometer of their character.

The single biggest predictor of children's resilience after a stressful experience is having safe, stable, and nurturing relationships and environments. Caregivers need to consistently show children that they are seen and that their needs matter. In practice, parents can do the following:

- **Seek out additional support from friends, family, schools, mental health professionals, or pediatricians.** While having many supports can be helpful, even one reliable source of unconditional support can make a big difference. Often the healthy siblings need to process and reflect on their experiences with a more neutral source than a parent.
- **Solicit and communicate about the experience of the sibling, imagining what their life would be like without their sibling's challenge.** Siblings want to please and protect their parents, so may not share difficult feelings without being invited to do so. Give unconditional support, provide space for them to have breaks from the extra responsibilities they may have, and prioritize their safety at all times (for example, if their sibling has violent behavioral problems).
- **Manage and set realistic expectations.** Sometimes when one child struggles, we expect more of other children in the home. Siblings can often rise to these expectations, but there are limits—toddlers have tantrums, older children and teens may still be developmentally oriented to think of themselves first, and sibling conflict should be expected even when one sibling is sick or struggling.
- **Engage siblings as caregiving partners when they are developmentally ready.** It's important to recognize their ability to contribute to the family, show them their involvement is appreciated, and leave room for the other parts of their childhood.
- **Make time for siblings.** For the siblings, try to remember that sometimes it may feel hard or unfair that they have less parental attention. Rather than feeling guilty about this reality, find ways to connect with the sibling to heal this gap.

For siblings of chronically or seriously ill children, they face the additional struggle of integrating this mixed experience into their identity. When I speak with families and professionals about this, the recurring theme is the catch-22 of being the "little helper."

When families have two children close in age, the older sibling is often encouraged to be involved in the younger child's care. By allowing the big sibling to be the "little helper" and grab a diaper or a bottle for the baby, you can keep the big sibling busy, engaged, and connected to family life. But of course, sometimes the big sibling may not want to be the "little helper." He may want to go to the park instead of sitting home during nap time, or maybe he wants his parents to himself for a while. This struggle can be real and lead to behavioral setbacks during the adjustment period.

For siblings of children with challenges, this dynamic is escalated in importance and intensity. When siblings see the importance of caregiving, they can feel the satisfaction and self-esteem of truly helping their loved one. It can be a deeply meaningful, positive experience that grounds them and affects the way that they think of themselves. But when being a "little helper" feels forced or overwhelms a child's other identities, it can lead to resentment and anger.

Sammy, one of my patients with epilepsy, was having a severe prolonged seizure at home with a babysitter who did not know what to do. His sister Lily, eight years old at the time, jumped into action. She got the medication out and called 911, despite having to hide in the pantry because the babysitter was crying so loudly, she couldn't hear the emergency dispatcher's instructions. For Lily, as she went through high school and considered her future, no single experience was likely similarly impactful. She felt like she saved her brother's life (and may have!) and by extension, she felt like a superhero. She's now a teenager and deciding among careers in the health-care industry, looking to match her strengths with a career where she could have a lifesaving impact.

I know dozens of doctors who were inspired to pursue their profession because of these sorts of experiences. In middle school, I was at a cheerleading sleepaway camp, and I had long and extremely active days. The littlest member of our squad, the one we threw up in the air for stunts, had type 1 diabetes. I'll never forget finding her just before bed completely disoriented. She had been twice as active, eaten half the food, and taken her normal insulin. She was in a hypoglycemic crisis. In hindsight, I did very little other than bring her altered state to the attention of the adults around me, but at the time I thought that if I hadn't said something, maybe she wouldn't have woken up in the morning. So, truly, I think these early positive experiences of caregiving can help build self-esteem.

The siblings of children with challenges see the world through a unique perspective, and many of them divide the world into two groups—people who get it and those who don't. Siblings often develop a strategy for who they tell and who they do not tell along these lines, and it's best to allow them to maintain this control whenever possible. It's helpful to let the teacher, principal, or school counselor know what your sibling is dealing with at home. Just as this is useful when the parents are getting a divorce or when the family is moving, the stress from home can show up at school and the school community will be better able to address this when they know what's going on at home.

Some children may also benefit from the ability to be in an environment where they can forget their additional responsibilities as the "little helper" and feel more typical. Spending time with their peers may be particularly important for this reason. For siblings, it's important that they are seen and valued for who they are outside of their identity as a caregiver. These siblings are loved unconditionally and valued when they contribute and when they do not.

If this is relevant to your situation, I encourage you to dig deep to bring as much compassion as you can to the situation. If a sibling expresses that they need a break, the parent may feel disappointed or frustrated. How can you need a break from your sibling? This can be particularly hard to hear if the caregiving parent feels inadequately supported and if they need a break too. But communication of this sort is an opportunity for parents to show siblings unconditional love. Their feelings and preferences matter. Children can love their siblings and value their families and still need space and balance in their lives.

Sometimes, children's honesty about these needs can inspire other family members to express mixed feelings. But when we show the siblings that they are unconditionally valued, we can remind ourselves that we are too.

In this chapter, we've discussed the importance of a co-caregiver and how to include other family members in the work you are doing to support your child through a challenge. Because some responsibilities feel more urgent, I have seen families underinvest the time necessary to enlist, train, and maintain these valued members of the care team. But when you have collaborators with whom you can have constructive, productive dialogues, it can be a huge help. We've also focused on the siblings who have their own needs and we've discussed how the experience of being a sibling is often a mixed blessing. Sometimes siblings can feel boxed in to being a helper or feel harmed by seeing family resources— time, money, or attention—being diverted away from their needs. But siblings can also learn and grow in response to this stress—gaining skills in empathy, resilience, and independence.

In the next chapter, we're going to focus on the developmental themes that affect your journey as a parent. While many assume bigger children are easier to parent through a challenge, it's not always so simple. As children gain skills, their needs also evolve, and while every child moves through these phases at their own pace, thinking through these trajectories can help you plan ahead. Before moving past this section, take a moment to reflect on the people closest to you and your child.

- If you have a co-parent, how is the balance of caregiving duties working for you? How is your communication style?
- Are there other resources in your inner or outer circle you could use for the benefit of your family?

- Are there reasons you hesitate to ask for help from the people who care for your family?
- If you have other children, how are they, really? What challenges do you anticipate them facing in the future, and how can you better support them?

CHAPTER 8

Respecting Your Child's Space and Development

In addition to being bald and fitted with an infusion port for my chemo-therapy treatments, I was also a very small kindergartener. My parents were nervous about sending me to a school where I was too small and weak to open the doors by myself. One day, a first grader pushed me to the ground and called me "baldy." I hopped up, yelled right back at them, and went about my day cheerful and content. But even in the '80s, this was promptly identified as unacceptable bullying behavior, and my parents, teachers, and the principal got involved. It was at this point that I began to feel mortified, ashamed, and resentful. I felt that I was strong enough to take care of myself and these adults were drawing attention to me in a way that just made me feel *less capable*.

As I grew older, things shifted. At eleven, I was a healthy and rela-tively independent *A* student, and nearly my adult height. Once, after a routine physical, I answered the phone and the caller, assuming I was my mother, said, "You need to bring Kelly in for more testing; some-thing came back abnormal." So, I asked more questions: "What was it and why is more testing needed?" The nurse on the other end said something along the lines of, "The cancer could be back." I didn't sleep that night and didn't tell my mother until the next day. I was terrified thinking my life might be over. Even once I knew it was a false alarm, I clung to the worry that my life could be ruined any time by a simple phone call.

As a spunky five-year-old, I felt my capacity was underestimated by those around me, but as a tween, I felt everyone assumed I was capable, when really I was more fragile than ever. As a pediatrician, I have seen these patterns recur with other children. We think of growth as a linear process, advancing from dependent to independent, but, as children develop a more complex inner life, sometimes they need even more support from their care team than they did as preschoolers.

We'll spend this chapter talking through some of the common considerations in parenting children of various stages and then further exploring the themes that apply to all children.

Special Considerations by Stage

As you think about crafting the ideal plan for your child, it's important to meet them where they are developmentally. While a child's priorities are intrinsically unique to the individual and their family, by understanding age-based trends we can communicate more effectively and anticipate what challenges our children face.

Bear in mind, these ranges are broad and subject to limitation. Not every child will hit all these stages or hit them on the same time line. We know that many children facing challenges have developmental delays or disabilities. Some kids will communicate in the style of a toddler well into their teen years, and that's part of who they are and potentially part of the unique parenting challenge. In the following section, I group children by developmental stage to discuss themes families face in parenting, and I risk reinforcing ableist norms and causing parents to feel shame about a child who may not fit the typical range of development. Please know that comparisons to healthy peers may not be fair or appropriate for your child, and your care team can help you with more specific advice tailored to your child. My hope is that by examining the trends in how children face challenges by stage, I can comment on some more specific strategies to help you build your caregiving plans around your child's current needs.

Babies and Toddlers

We expect children aged three and younger to be fully dependent upon us. We know they need help sleeping, feeding, and interacting with their environment; when they have extra needs, it doesn't feel so out of the ordinary. Children who are this age developmentally often cannot discuss the issues at hand, but these children still have preferences and needs that should be respected.

Commonly, these preferences tend to revolve around the child's schedule. Few things have more profound impacts on a child's behavior and growth and the family well-being than sleep. Appointments, disruptive symptoms, or care requirements that interrupt sleep should all be minimized when possible. In addition to hours spent sleeping, I find we're often quick to forget that children at this stage need free time and the opportunity to play to promote their development. Too often, I have seen a child with some developmental delays end up with restricted play time and extra time restrained in a car seat or stroller due to the demands of appointments. To advocate for our children, we have to protect their right to rest and to play.

When it comes to communicating with children of this age, their abilities are frequently underestimated. Expressive communication develops before verbal speech. Behavior and gaze are valuable indicators of a child's thoughts and preferences. Even when a child cannot speak, a parent can observe what they like and dislike. Whether you are trying to troubleshoot through a typical parenting struggle or an extra caregiving demand, using your observations can help. Frequently, toddlers demand control and fight restraint—even the restraint of a high chair or being held in place to have their teeth brushed—vigorously. Many parents observe that standing diaper changes are easier than forcing their kid to recline on a changing table. Similarly holding a child still to administer an inhaled medication may be more difficult and traumatic than bringing the medication to them when they are distracted and busy at play even if it means you lose some control and end up chasing your child around as they play.

Janet Lansbury, parenting expert and author of *Elevating Child Care*, asserts that infants and toddlers deserve to be treated as intrinsically capable people from day one. Lansbury advocates for informing children about anything relevant to their lives with clear, honest, and direct communication, and I tend to agree. While it might feel weird to tell a nine-month-old, "Now it's time for your daily medication," when you know they are likely to respond, "Baa baa na na," I do recommend you talk to your child about their care, no matter how young they are.

There are also benefits to building trust and routines. By communicating, "Now it's time for your medicine," you give your child a moment to anticipate and prepare. In addition, when you say it, your body language and facial expressions have a chance to set the tone. Even if your child cannot hear you, children are often incredibly perceptive to these nonverbal communication cues and may be more likely to participate productively. In the context of your relationship, saying firmly and clearly, "Now we need to do this and it's important," is essential if it's something your child doesn't enjoy.

When communicating with this age group, it's important not to let the communication escalate to an argument. Not only will you lose, but you will also likely end up frustrated. My children both had frequent ear infections and hated taking antibiotics. I would tell them, "It's time," and give them a choice to drink the medication from a cup or take it from a syringe. If they started fighting it, I would choose and give the medication to a kicking and screaming toddler. Then I'd give them a hug and say, "You really didn't like that, but the next time will be better." Sure enough, by the third or fourth time, they would drink the medication without crying.

Of course, seeing the tantrum begin, it's tempting to try to comfort them and postpone giving the medication. But when you begin down this pathway, you give the child the impression that they have all the power and can choose to take the medication or not. We know that most children do not have a choice, though finding a way to give a child a sense of control or agency in the process can be helpful. Sometimes they can choose when, where, or how a medication is administered. But once you have decided it's time, it's time.

Clarity and strong parental leadership will, over time, provide a sense of safety and predictability for your child. Though this may be more forceful in some ways, it's also kinder to your child because they know what to expect and will feel safer. Being firm will also decrease the anticipatory anxiety that is sometimes worse than the actual activity.

Preschoolers

In the preschool years, we see more emerging capability, and allowing your child to participate in their care can make things easier. Children can surprise us with their abilities. I remember watching a three-year-old with type 1 diabetes stick her own finger with a lancet and use a glucometer to check her blood sugar. She had mastered this complex task and demonstrated maturity about using a needle on her own finger at an age when many children hadn't yet learned to use a toilet because she had so many opportunities to practice.

At this stage, children's communication skills are advancing and often children ask a lot of questions, the sort that can confuse, upset, or stump their caregivers. Although their thirst for knowledge has expanded, their ability to fully understand complex situations is highly variable. Sometimes they will surprise you with their sophisticated understanding, and other times they will astound you with their ability to misunderstand reality.

Precisely because imaginations are so vivid at this age, sharing information with your child is important. Giving your child concrete facts about their situation will help them feel safe and help establish open communication. Prioritizing honesty in your communication will facilitate trust and healthy attachment. If they ask if something will hurt, you can be honest and help them put the pain in context by explaining, "It will hurt, but it will be over by the time you count to three," or, "It will hurt, but the doctors will be giving you medicine to help it hurt less." You can also make a plan for coping together when you can anticipate what's coming. You can tell your child, "If it hurts, you can grab my hand or say, 'Ouch.'"

Many parents feel confused about how to know what's developmentally appropriate to share. In this preschool stage, children live in the here and now. Sharing information about something that is more than a few days away is not often helpful. If you are notably sad and worried because in three months your child will have to have a surgery, you can share that you are feeling sad and worried, but you can protect them from having to think and talk about a surgery three months away. When you do want to talk to them about the surgery, probably no more than a week before it happens, you can prepare yourself as much as possible to go into that conversation feeling calm. You should also anticipate that they will want to know the practical details of what they will experience.

You can learn a lot from your care team, teachers, and other parents about how they talk to children about their challenges. Explaining things to a child is a difficult task and takes both a sophisticated understanding of what children face and a nuanced understanding of the child's cognitive development. When they ask questions and you don't know how to respond, admit it. You can simply say that it's a good question and you need time to think about it, or to do some research, or to ask someone on your care team before you can respond.

Often children this age will get "stuck" on one feature of their lives, something that was unexpected, scary, or notable. It could be that they saw a green taxi and all other taxis they have seen are yellow. A child might remember and ask about something like this for weeks or even months. This remains true of children facing challenges—they may remember and remind you of the day you forgot their braces or the day they rode in an ambulance. While this may be a signal of a trauma, it may also be their way of processing a novel experience. Allowing the child to talk through those noteworthy experiences, acting them out with stuffed animals, or drawing pictures of them, can sometimes help the child find peace.

Six- to Eleven-Year-Olds

From ages six to ten, we see children's worlds expand. They enter school and their needs for independence, for privacy, and to be listened to become more pressing. At this age, children have a high capacity to master new tasks and will often feel delight in doing so, but still require supervision as they lack the maturity to be dependable. Children this age can tell you what's important to them and often don't hesitate to do so, loudly.

Sometimes, the things children want at this age are harder to substitute. A parent can't play the same way a friend can. Kicking a soccer ball around with a parent can't compare to the experience of being on a team. The increasing complexity of their needs can make it more difficult for caregivers to center plans around them. Additionally, the volatility of their needs can be hard to anticipate. In one month, the world may begin and end with a specific friendship, and by the next, it may be an entirely different relationship that matters. There isn't always a rhyme or reason to these changes.

Because children begin to show more trust and interest in others outside of the family, often they seek sources of information other than their parents. Anticipating this need for third-party information and verification can help you support their needs. On the way to a follow-up appointment, encourage them to think up a question. When they are allowed screen time, at some point show them a website with appropriate information that might interest them.

It's important for all children to have safe, stable, and nurturing relationships to promote their mental health. Children who are facing challenges may need even more support. Parents can help by finding and facilitating relationships with trusted individuals, whether at school or any number of community organizations (like a sports team, church, or volunteer group). Fortifying this support before a crisis arises, or before the hormones and drama of puberty arrive, can be helpful. The more close support your child has, the more likely they are to reach out and get the help they need, even when sometimes they may prefer that their support comes from someone other than their parent.

Tweens and Teens

In some ways, the late tween and teen years make things a bit easier. By this point, a child's abilities and communication skills allow them to drive their care and take over tasks, like communicating with a teacher or stopping at the pharmacy to pick up a refill independently. Some children of this age can begin to "own" the responsibility of prioritizing their own medical or educational needs. However, these years can be some of the most challenging stages, both for the child and the caregiver.

Children at this age often need and value the opinions and ideas of their peers more than their parents. Sometimes they can resist doing the right thing for their health because they demand their independence and need to assert their identity as separate from their parents. Some teens also demand privacy and refuse to be cared for, even when they need it.

Though they may be adult sized, their judgment and the ability to make good decisions has not reached full maturity. They may struggle with considering the long- and short-term consequences of their decisions, including their health decisions. Their decision-making won't be fully developed until their late teens, early twenties, or even later. And the hormonal volatility of puberty doesn't help.

Transitioning a child to fully managing their condition as an adult is a complex process and has been the focus of a lot of research in the past few years.[1] Consensus seems to be that the process takes about ten years. This may cause you to raise your eyebrows. Ten years is half of childhood, or the entirety of the teenage years. Because this transition is so important to your child's well-being, you should seek help in the process from your care team.

While you allow your child more and more responsibility, a parent has to learn to let go. In parenting a teen, the goal is that they make all the decisions. To get to that point requires a parent to give up control and develop trust and faith in their child. A parent's role might transition to that of a mentor or a coach. Instead of solving problems you see, you help children learn to identify problems and troubleshoot in their own way.

Inevitably during this transition, children make mistakes. From the outside, it's so obvious; of course, mistakes are part of learning. But when you watch your own child jeopardize their health in some way by not making a good choice, it can be terrifying and upsetting. From this perspective, parents may wonder what they've done wrong, how they can fix it, and if their child will ever achieve independence. It's important to remember that you aren't in this process alone. Everyone on the care team—teachers, doctors, therapists, coaches, family, faith leaders, and neighbors—are there to support you in this transition.

Like the other transitions inherent to childhood—learning to sleep, for example—it's two steps forward, one step back. Development is a trend, and it's not always predictable. Having a firm understanding of what our children are developmentally capable of can guide our parenting and our caregiving. But some of the strategies for respecting your child transcend age and development.

Universal Parenting Tensions

While parenting a two-year-old through a challenge feels intrinsically very different than parenting a teen through a challenge, several parenting dilemmas are universally present. Setting limits, establishing healthy communication, sparing our children difficulties when we can, and allowing them input and control are core parts of parenting that become trickier when your family faces a challenge.

Setting Firm, Consistent, and Empathetic Limits

All parents struggle with setting limits. Imagine a parent whose elementary school child is struggling to fall and stay asleep. The parent can choose whether to extend the bedtime or allow them to sleep in the parent's bed. When that child is on long-term cancer treatments, with medications that make sleep more difficult, can a parent still make those choices? Parents whose children require caregiving often have a harder time setting and keeping limits firm. When our children are facing challenges, we feel for them and want to lessen their load as much as possible. A caregiving parent may hesitate to say no when their child asks for nonnutritious food for dinner when it's not on the menu—when your child has been through a lot, it can feel difficult to impose a rule, or even consequence, for example, when they misbehave. But children still need structure even when they are unwell.

Discipline—the process of teaching your child how to behave and what's right and wrong—is still essential. Parents know their children better than anyone and often can instinctively know where boundaries should be, but when a child is suffering, we all want to be more flexible. Caregiving parents sometimes feel ambivalent, sad, or anxious when children have to tolerate procedures or therapy regimens that are uncomfortable. Providing extra comfort and love in these settings is natural and best for your child. For the two weeks after a surgery, maybe extra ice cream, more screen time, and a more flexible bedtime make sense. But in the big picture, limits can help set a child up for success.

When children have limits, the predictability promotes feelings of safety. Boundaries can help children regulate their behavior and emotions. However, when a child's life is not following a typical trajectory, discipline feels more complicated. A parent may be uncertain about what an appropriate boundary is. When is the appropriate time to potty train your child if they have developmental delays or disabilities, or if they take medications that affect their voiding and stooling? After a medical trauma like a surgery or hospitalization, children may need time to readjust to their normal routine, but how long—days or weeks? When a child is going through a tough time, of course they will act out more, but when do you tolerate the behavior and when do you intervene?

When it comes to identifying appropriate boundaries and expectations for your child, don't hesitate to speak with others on your care team who may have insights. While doctors, nurses, teachers, and parents have likely seen other children in situations similar to your child, they may not have all the answers. Sometimes they can be a great sounding board as you find the line for your family, and the process of discussing the situation can help you gain confidence in your choice. When setting limits and expectations for your child, remember that you are the expert on your child. Keep these tips in mind when setting limits:

- When changing the rules, try to keep it simple. Changing one thing (e.g., "This week we will work on sitting at the table for meals") at a time increases the likelihood you will see success.
- Inform everyone in your home of the new expectation, consider posting the rules, and be precise: "Now that Bobby has had a few days to recover from his surgery, we're going back to the rules from before—only one TV show a day."
- Sometimes you don't know how your child will react until you try. A new rule can result in a short period of "testing" or bad behavior, and a real try can mean committing to something for a few days before you know if the new plan is working.
- Be firm. When you feel ambivalent about the plan, sometimes that adds to confusion and reduces the likelihood of the limit working.
- Sometimes you may institute a rule that does not go well. Give yourself grace and remember that you can change your mind and try other techniques.
- Even when a child is suffering, sick, or in pain, if your child is hitting, biting, or physically harming others, it's important to set limits to protect everyone.

Setting expectations, limits, and rules is part of parenting, but often it can be confusing. In my experience, parental intuition can be really helpful as you make these decisions.

Maintaining Open Communication

Parents often prepare for big talks with their children. A family has just gotten a new diagnosis of inflammatory bowel disease, and now the family will pick a day to sit down, inform the children about the diagnosis, and explain how the treatment plan will change life over the next few months. These big, intentional talks may help start conversations but deliver only a small percentage of the actionable information and support your family needs.

Just as it's a process for caregiving parents to accept information and learn, children also need time to do this. We know that adults can only absorb between 40 and 80 percent of what they are told in a doctor's visit.[2] Children likely process less, especially if they do not perceive the information as important or understand the context. Because of this, no matter how excellent your big talks are, you should expect that questions and learning will continue over time. A child progresses in their understanding, their condition evolves, and the plan changes, and all of this necessitates more communication. To make matters even more complex, the child also develops and changes their capabilities over time. Even when things improve, a child will look back and ask questions to help understand what they went through.

To facilitate open communication, it's a good idea to build in regular opportunities to talk about the challenge and about other parts of everyday life too. Not only does this regular communication inform your family, but it also helps foster connection. Some families use a daily check-in to share what were the best and worst parts of the day. Other families might use a family meeting every week to go over the parts of their life that matter, from logistics to goal-setting. Some children open up when relaxing before bed or on the drive commuting to school.

These check-ins provide opportunities for children to be reminded of upcoming events and ask questions. You can share the idea that all feelings and ideas are welcome. Parents can model goal-setting, problem-solving, and asking for help. Communication can increase cohesion within your family and make you feel more like a team.[3]

For children who are not verbal, it's still essential to maximize their capacity for communication. Augmentative alternative communication systems—including low-tech solutions like pointing to a picture on a communication board or higher-tech options like a speech-generating device—can improve overall quality of life and participation in family meetings.

Functional communication with your child can also facilitate task management. When you are delegating tasks, sometimes it's easy to feel fatigued by nagging individuals who may not always listen. But mixing up your style, communicating with humor or with writing, can help you catch the attention of your family members and maybe promote their listening. If you're trying to help your child learn to take their medication on their own without a reminder, you can put a stop sign with a picture of a pill bottle on the door and point to it when leaving the house. One day when they forget, you can make a joke out of it and pretend to be the medicine bottle and say, "Oh no, you forgot about me," and pretend to cry.[4] Humor and playfulness can help relieve all kinds of family tension and improve communication, including a family facing a challenge.

A Positive Communication Strategy

Nicole was a nine-year-old with anxiety and dyslexia. Sometimes talking about her conditions seemed to make things worse. When her mother discussed this with me, I reflected back the way she would talk about her daughter's conditions. The mother described how Nicole found her "intrusive, uncontrollable anxiety" upsetting, and her "failure to learn to read" was interfering not just with academics but also with her ability to make and keep friends at school.

Together we reflected on the power of words. Nicole's mom had been so busy balancing all the caregiving demands and raising her other children, she had not reflected on how she spoke about her daughter's challenge. The words she used were correct and described Nicole, but they also emphasized the conditions as fixed and negative.

We wondered together if she might rebrand these issues at the next discussion. We brainstormed how we could explain to Nicole that her brain works differently, just like every brain does. Some parts of her brain might make her life better and easier like her creativity or her attention to detail, but some parts might mean she has to work harder at things. Luckily, she had her mom, her doctors, and her teachers by her side to help her figure things out.

Children deserve honesty. When a parent speaks to a child disingenuously about their condition, this may compromise trust and attachment in the long run. When a parent instead intentionally chooses ways to focus on a child's power over the condition, the strength of the child's support network, and the hope for improvement over time, this can change the tone of how a child sees their condition. When you are able to point out their strengths and advantages as you discuss their challenges, you can remind children of their inherent capability.

Sparing Children Our Difficulties When We Can

A mother is understandably very anxious and stressed about her child's upcoming blood draw. Perhaps she is sensitive to needles herself and experiences with her other children having blood work were traumatic for her. The mother may talk about the blood draw a lot with the child and others, seeking support. When they walk into the room where the procedure is to be done, the mother's body language may be uncertain and her tone of voice with the phlebotomist is questioning. The child picks up on Mom's fears and skepticism and becomes anxious and hesitant, too, resisting the procedure because of fear. While the child probably would have worried and cried anyway, the mother's way of coping with the stress made the situation worse.

I've seen this scenario play out many times, and I want to emphasize that I've been on the parent side of this too when my children have had general anesthesia for surgeries. The anxiety and distress you feel when your child is going into a procedure can feel enormous and unavoidable. Only a robot could walk into some of these situations without stress. Some children are very sensitive and perceptive of a parent's stress. We can't always control our stress level, but we can control when a child is informed about things, the actions we take, and the words we use.

Parents can exercise mindfulness and check in with themselves during these stressful moments. This can give you the opportunity to choose how you respond with intention. You can take a moment to ask yourself if your behavior is helping or hurting your child. You should particularly consider your body language and rapport with the phlebotomist, doctor, or surgeon, as your child is watching. If you show your child that you know them and trust them, this can meaningfully decrease the anxiety your child feels about the novel situation.

If you want to talk to the doctor about something the child may find upsetting, you can try to do so over the phone or while a nurse or secretary in the doctor's office sits with your child. While you may have weeks of anticipation before a surgery, likely a young child doesn't need to know or worry for weeks because we can protect them from this prolonged anticipation. Often as a parent, you have an opportunity and a responsibility to set the tone for your family. When you feel overwhelmed by what you face as a caregiving parent, when you are able to cope with that stress, you'll set your child up for success.

Allowing Your Children Input and Control

Giving children choice helps them feel like they have power and control. Children tend to be happier and often gain confidence with practice making good decisions. Because children who face challenges often have more things they *have to do*, choice can be even more appealing and empowering. The entire caregiving plan is designed to help your child and affects your schedule as a parent, but it's their future, it's their body, and it's their growth and development, so of course they deserve to be a central part of the decisions about their health.

While this sounds obvious, when things get busy, caregivers have little time, patience, or energy to devote to this goal. Medical and educational systems aren't always designed to incorporate input from children. How can we allow children input?

Consider Nella, a six-year-old girl with unclear speech. After a few years of hoping she might grow out of it, the pediatricians and educators have agreed it's time for speech therapy. The caregiving parent decides that speech therapy is not optional—it has to happen even if Nella doesn't want it, because it's for her benefit. Still, the plan to execute therapy might take Nella's perspective into account. Would she prefer teletherapy or in person? Would she prefer to practice her exercises with Mom or Dad? Would she like to pick a prize, like a special movie or book, after she has done it for a month? Some more sophisticated children will have the interest and ability to dig in on all these decisions, but some children starting out may feel overwhelmed by too much choice and control. As a parent, you know your child's personality and preferences, so you can best navigate this balance.

Children who are unable to cognitively and verbally engage in these discussions can still express their feelings. A child may show you with their behavior and expressions what they prefer. Sometimes caregiving parents have to be the ones to translate and help advocate for these preferences.

We know that as children grow, their needs evolve. Many parents feel that as soon as they figure out a stage of parenting and find a rhythm, something changes. Considering where your child is in their developmental progression can help us predict and prepare to meet their needs and adapt our parenting strategies. Setting limits, communicating with your child, and promoting their independence are important parenting goals for all children, even when they face a challenge.

In the next part, we'll discuss coping with some of the difficult emotions that accompany facing a challenge. We will begin by considering how part of being an effective caregiver is confronting some difficult feelings. While these are sensitive topics not often shared in public circles, many if not most parents confront feelings of grief, guilt, anxiety, anger, and shame at some point. We'll talk about coping with these feelings and when to consider getting extra support.

Before you move on from this chapter, think about some important considerations:

- Consider what stage your child fits in and what needs are most prominent.
- Reflect on your limits; do they feel too lax, too strict, or just right?
- Think about your communication frequency and the underlying tone.
- Imagine things from your child's perspective; can you find ways to incorporate their preferences into their care?

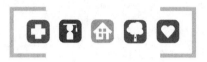

PART III

MANAGING EMOTIONS

CHAPTER 9

Confronting Hard Feelings and Burnout

Derrick was a ten-year-old boy who had been struggling in school. Despite tutors and extra parental investment in his schooling, things were harder than they should have been. His parents sought out evaluations in hopes of finding a better path forward for their son. These evaluations found that their son did not have specific learning disabilities or an underlying condition like ADHD. However, the testing did reveal that his intelligence or IQ was lower than expected.

Although the results didn't indicate a disability, for this family, it was disappointing news. The family had hoped the problem was one that could clearly be solved. If he had a learning disability, he could benefit from an educational intervention. If he had ADHD, he could take medication. But instead, the family was left with a bigger challenge: acceptance.

When I chatted with Derrick's mother about it, I asked if she thought her own IQ might be similarly low. She started to cry. She confided that, yes, she did think her son's IQ and educational challenges were very similar to what she herself had experienced growing up. She felt guilty. She wanted to give her son every advantage and not pass on what she saw as a liability.

When we dug deeper into her history and her experience growing up with a lower-than-average IQ, it became clear that the most difficult thing was not the IQ itself; it was that those around her had not understood it. Her accomplishments were compared to others with different strengths, and important people in her life often saw her as coming up short. Her teachers and parents had labeled her as lazy, when she was really trying her best. When she was growing up, the path to success seemed so narrow: good grades, high test scores, and entry to prestigious schools.

She felt bad. Derrick's mother struggled to process her feelings—she felt sad, guilty, angry, and worried. As I struggled with how to best support her in this challenging parenting moment, I reminded her that she was the perfect parent for her son. I told her that everything she had learned from her experience could help her to help her son. She knew her son's capacities, and so she could choose to focus on her son's work effort and growth, rather than comparing his test scores to those of her peers.

Her family could choose to highlight and lean in to her son's strengths. They could help him find activities that would allow his exceptional social and emotional skills, his caring nature, and his athleticism to shine. They could stress that those talents would open a lot of pathways to a fulfilling life and that he is perfect just the way he is. Together, they could help their son select goals that made the most sense for his skills and strengths. In the end, this knowledge was a gift that would enable them to advocate for their son.

When working with families who are coming to grips with a difficult truth, be it a disability or a diagnosis, I've often relied on a positive pivot: "I know it's hard, but now that we have this information, we can do better." We can't always fix the root cause, but we can modify the environment and our own expectations to improve the outcome.

This begins with understanding that, no matter your child's challenge, it is not your fault. Our difficulties and our "weaknesses" as individuals make us who we are, as much as our strengths. While we have a tendency to look for the root cause so that we can "fix" it, sometimes we have to acknowledge and accept that things are just the way they are.

We have the most control over ourselves: our feelings and reactions to the challenge we're facing. Most parents, when facing a lot of stress, feel terrible. And it's not easy to know how to feel better when you feel bad. But I encourage parents to take their own feelings seriously, so that we can not only care for ourselves, but be better equipped to care for our children. When you know why you are feeling bad, you can make a plan to feel better. When you explore why you are feeling bad, even if you can't fix that feeling, understanding where it's coming from will help you.

When I counsel children about anxiety and sadness, I often use the analogy of a cloud. It's okay and expected to feel rained on or in a dark place, but when you have the deep understanding that those feelings will pass, it can help you endure the tough times. This analogy also helps to remind children that feeling bad doesn't make them bad. Even amidst tough times, they are always surrounded by people who love them.

In the following sections, we'll explore the negative feelings many parents experience when their children face challenges. While many of these topics are sensitive and uncomfortable to consider, it's necessary to explore them. Precisely because they are so difficult and some carry stigma, I've found that parents frequently feel alone and as if they cannot talk to anyone about this. Many parents try to tough it out alone, but glossing over or ignoring these hard topics will not make them go away.

Sadness and Grief

As parents, it's difficult for us to witness our children experiencing hardships. It could be your challenge is something more temporary, such as appendicitis or a broken bone, and seeing your child ill can make you feel sad, but generally speaking this type of challenge is easier to recover from. Others may have a child with a disability or a child with a physical or mental health diagnosis expected to be long-term. Still more families may have expected to have a child with certain attributes—athleticism, intelligence, good looks, or a certain gender—and ended up with the child they have instead.

For these families, you may have envisioned your child's life—and your life—one way, and now you have to adjust your expectations. You had dreams and ambitions about your child's future and what that would be like—sports they might play, schools they might attend, and the relationship you might have with them. And now, in coping with this diagnosis, you have to reset your expectations and change your plans.

In "Welcome to Holland," Emily Perl Kingsley's seminal essay about raising a differently abled child, the author uses the analogy of planning a family trip to Italy, reading guidebooks, and developing a plan for their visit...only to step off the flight and find themselves in Holland.

There is nothing wrong with Holland; it has tulips and Rembrandts. But it doesn't have gondolas and the Leaning Tower of Pisa. But everyone else seems to be traveling to Italy, leading to feelings of isolation. The change in plans is a disappointment and one over which you had no control or method of remediation.

Kingsley wrote the essay acknowledging the grief that accompanied facing the unexpected challenge of her child's diagnosis of trisomy 21 (commonly referred to as Down syndrome). However, she ends with the idea that, despite grieving the fact that she did not go to Italy, she found joy in Holland. We can find joy in our children for who they are, no matter what diagnosis they carry.[1]

Sometimes difficult diagnoses come with unexpected opportunities for joy. For example, children with a genetic disorder called Williams syndrome can have serious heart disease, difficulty growing, and developmental delays. These associated features can range in severity but do bring hardship: some may have severe learning difficulties and most have congenital heart disease—supravalvular aortic stenosis—which can require hospitalization and surgery. However, children with Williams syndrome also have a unique affinity for music and tend to be extremely social—personality features that can bring a lot of joy to those around them.

We need to remind ourselves that a child is more than their diagnosis. Every person—diagnosis or not—has strengths and difficulties, and things that come easily or provide challenges. Never have I thought,

"I'm so glad I had childhood cancer and the health complications that followed." However, I acknowledge that the experience is part of who I am. I am thankful for the role models I met and the lessons I learned by being a patient.

Focusing on the positives and cultivating gratitude is one strategy to cope with sadness from a difficult diagnosis. But many parents jump right to this step without giving themselves grace. When facing a change of plans, grief is expected—especially if your children may carry diagnoses that bring pain, risk, hardship, and loss. A parent will often need to grieve the loss of the healthy childhood they had envisioned for their child. Parents may feel stigma with the simple act of feeling sad or disappointed, but grieving does not mean that you do not love your child just the way they are. Sometimes giving yourself permission to be sad allows you to find your way to coping.

In pediatrics, we often tout the resilience of children. Children bounce back in a way that's downright miraculous. But many physicians who have worked with parents after their children face hardships have seen how incredibly resilient parents can be too.

Models for Moving through Grief

The sad part of parenthood isn't well publicized. Elizabeth Stone, an educator and author of several parenting books, once said that to be a parent is to "decide forever to have your heart go walking around outside your body." Parenthood makes us uniquely vulnerable. Inconveniences that may seem minor when they happen to someone else can seem major when they happen to your child. Because we think of children as healthy and happy, when their lives are anything less than perfect it can feel like a deep betrayal.

Although famed psychiatrist Elisabeth Kübler-Ross later remodeled and expanded on her well-known grief model, for our purposes, her initial five stages of grief can be helpful. Parents regularly walk this path—going through denial, anger, bargaining, depression, and acceptance.

When we view grief through this lens, we can understand it as a process, rather than a static state. This framework can help some parents feel less stuck in their grief.

Other models of grief encourage us to take more ownership over our recovery. William Worden's four tasks of mourning describe the process of "driving our way through grief." Worden suggests we can work to accept our new reality, acknowledge our feelings, adjust to our new environment, and reinvest in our new life. When you are ready for it, a road map like this can help you to feel prepared to plot a way to feeling better. There is strength in acknowledging and accepting all of the intense feelings we will experience while caretaking our children.

The Way Things Used to Be

You will undoubtedly experience feelings of grief and sadness directly related to your child's challenges—seeing a child suffer is difficult. But some of your feelings may be about you. Many parents grieve the part of their life that has been edged out by new caregiving duties. Caregiving parents are nearly thirty times more likely to leave the workforce. They often spend several hours a week on care coordination, and frequently spend twenty hours a week more than typical parents giving their children direct care.[2] To feel disappointed or overwhelmed by this is expected and doesn't mean you are less of a parent.

I worked with a mother who had unexpectedly given up a successful and promising career to care for her child, who was diagnosed with heart disease and developmental disabilities. For this family it was not an intentional choice. The little boy had been diagnosed with his congenital heart defect after birth, while Mom was on maternity leave. Since Dad was working as they watched medical bills accumulate when a lot of his care needs began, Mom had been there to learn from the physical therapists and speak with the cardiologist. The next thing they knew, she was not returning to work.

She knew it was the right decision for her family. If she could go back, she would make the same decision intentionally. But she had been extremely thoughtful and intentional in her life plan and suddenly lost her sense of agency and control. There were times when she felt disappointed and frustrated. She would not be able to maximize her potential in her career of choice due to this new caregiving responsibility. Although her choice was right for her family, and it was consistent with her values and priorities, it still came at a cost. She resented how his father had a safe space at work where he could take a break from the difficulties of being home with a sick child. While their marriage was complicated, this resentment was one factor that likely led to their divorce.

She loved spending time with her son and preferred to be the one managing his day-to-day care, but she still grieved the loss of her career—the intellectual stimulation, office friends, and the positive self-regard that came from doing something she was very good at. You don't have to dislike the work of caregiving, you may enjoy it immensely, but you may also miss what you had before, whether it was more time for your job, your friends, your children, or yourself.

When people know you have a child who has been sick or struggling and ask how you are doing, it may feel selfish to say, "I miss my job," or, "I miss the rhythm our life had before I took on all of this extra responsibility." But you are allowed to feel however you feel. You can love your child immensely and still dislike some aspects of parenting. If the people around you judge you or make you feel like a lesser parent, it's likely because they lack the ability to understand and empathize with your situation. Being honest about how you are feeling can help you feel better, and it can help those around you support you more robustly. Had this mother, resentful about staying home, been able to communicate with her partner, perhaps they could have worked to find other solutions. Moreso, being honest about the mixed nature of your feelings may help build the empathy and understanding within your community to break through this stigma.

If your friends and family don't seem to understand this, you can look to parents who have children with unexpected needs and may get you. Several memoirs highlight these themes. *Catastrophic Rupture* recounts the story of a mother, a pediatric intensive care physician and ethicist, who had a traumatic birth and a daughter with a brain injury. Heather Lanier shares the story of her daughter with a rare genetic syndrome in *Raising a Rare Girl*. Therapy is another safe space where you can find help accepting all of your feelings.

Guilt

In addition to their sadness, many parents feel intense guilt when their child struggles. We know that we can't keep our children from experiencing hardships, but even so, most parents at one time or another have seen their child struggle and thought, "I should have protected them from this." Parents know these thoughts aren't rational, but that logic doesn't reduce our deep desire for the power to protect our children from struggles.

In most cases, the cause of the child's suffering was out of parental control, or the result of multiple factors. Consider:

- An older mom who has a baby with a trisomy 21 might feel it's her fault for choosing to get pregnant at an age with an increased risk for genetic abnormalities.
- Another parent might have a child who was injured in an accident at day care. The parent jumps to assuming the accident could have been prevented, and that it was his fault for not selecting a day care with better supervision.
- A child is diagnosed with inflammatory bowel disease after years of slow growth. The father worries the delayed diagnosis was his fault—if he had just pushed for a specialist sooner maybe the child would have gotten treatment sooner.

Let's unpack each of these cases. For the older mom, the difference in risk if she had gotten pregnant just five years earlier sounds substantial.

From the ages of thirty-five to forty, the risk changes from one case of trisomy 21 per 350 births to one case occurring per 95 births. However, when seen the other way, even in the higher-risk age group, the vast majority of births—more than 98 percent—still don't result in trisomy 21. Five years ago, you may not have been ready to have a child, emotionally or financially, or you may not have been in the same relationship. For that matter, five years ago you may still have given birth to a child with trisomy 21. Note too that older sperm is also known to affect the risk of various conditions, including autism, leukemia, schizophrenia, and birth defects, though the added risk of age may be more subtle. Parents should acknowledge that while our behaviors sometimes increase or decrease risk, there are other matters outside our control, like randomness and chance that result in our biological destiny. Lastly, while you may have "given" your child a genetic road map associated with hardship, you have also given your child life and the opportunity for a rich life as well, though it may differ from the life you envisioned.

For the case of an accident at a day care: Imagine the top of a slide, too many toddlers pushing to go in front, and one toppled over the railing, breaking his arm. The fall required a surgery and four weeks in a cast, but the child is expected to make a full recovery. Parents may jump to assign blame—the day care wasn't supervising sufficiently or maybe one parent chose the day care and the accident is their fault, accordingly. But again, random chance often has more to do with accidents than we'd like to acknowledge. Even the most vigilant care providers have situations where they are surprised, or multiple opportunities collide to result in an accident. It is important to analyze the situation to learn from it and to prevent another accident, but the analysis often doesn't do much for the child and family who has experienced the harm.

In the case where the child had slow growth for years and was ultimately diagnosed with inflammatory bowel disease, a parent might believe the pediatrician was negligent and should have gotten their child a diagnosis and specialized care earlier. However, many autoimmune or rare conditions have a long lead time prior to diagnosis. It may take years to reach an accurate assessment. It's unfair for a parent to think the issue could have been solved earlier because of the slow and subtle nature of some conditions. If the parent had taken the child to the gastroenterologist earlier, the child may not have been behind on growth enough to justify the invasive workup with sedation and colonoscopy required to make the diagnosis. It's not clear that the child would have been appropriately diagnosed and started on disease-modifying treatment earlier. It could be that the gastroenterologist would have said, "Let's see how the child grows over the next six to twelve months."

We have to acknowledge that guilt can sometimes be legitimate— even the best parents make mistakes, and there are accidents that can have serious repercussions and provide a reason for regret. For example, if a parent fell asleep holding their baby and the baby fell and sustained an injury, the parent might fixate on feelings of guilt. But we forget that the reason the parent was so tired in the first place was due to their efforts to care for the baby. We forget that every other day the parent had done everything right, and this one time they made a mistake and a split-second accident occurred. Whenever you consider your culpability for what your child is facing, consider how others would see it too, or what advice you would give a friend in your shoes.

How Guilt Creates Stress

All the logic in the world can't always chase away a parent's feelings of guilt. However, finding a way to confront the guilt is important for helping your child and for protecting your well-being as a caregiver. Guilt can be a toxic stressor that disrupts our body's balance.

Scientists have investigated the cumulative burden of chronic stress and life events on health outcomes. They call this kind of stress one's allostatic load, and when it exceeds our ability to cope, we begin to see many different conditions arise, including heart disease, cancer, diabetes, osteoporosis, neurological injury, and periodontal disease.[3]

Guilt is an intangible feeling that is difficult for doctors to biologically measure. At the same time, guilt has a significant impact on our body's physiological balance. When tragedy strikes our family, we can process this external stress as a traumatic event. Our guilt is an internal stressor, but excessive worrying can still be interpreted by the brain as a physical threat and cause harm due to physiological changes like reduced sleep quantity and quality and increased blood pressure and heart rate. While some worrying as discussed earlier is helpful, necessary, and constructive, excessive or invasive worrying can do more harm than good.

When parents take time to cope with these difficult feelings, they can improve their well-being as caregivers. One of the priorities in this book is to help you learn to cope and design a plan that is more sustainable for supporting your own health in addition to the health of your child. Some strategies include exploring the source of your guilt and naming it. Just saying out loud to yourself or someone else, "I feel guilty about my child's diagnosis," can be therapeutic. This statement can give you some distance from the feeling and some perspective. You can also reduce the burden by being kind to yourself and forgiving yourself.

Some parents have found another strategy to be helpful: They channel their guilt into a motivation for their advocacy work. Some families have focused their energy toward sharing knowledge with others to prevent the same confusion, suffering, or similar injuries. Most nonprofit work, including incredibly impactful organizations like Moms Demand Action (to reduce gun violence), National Alliance on Mental Illness, Alex's Lemonade Stand, and hundreds of others were started by individuals who were motivated to make change. Parents often find that taking action and doing something about those difficult feelings can help. The process of doing something can also build community and help you process what you are going through.

Fear and Anxiety

Two good friends of mine recently had their first baby. They were delighted by the experience. The social media pictures were "Pinterest perfect." However, as a close friend, I knew this baby was a medical miracle, helped along by years of effort, loss, and professional intervention. But the parents were rightfully overjoyed—everything was going great, from breastfeeding to sleeping. They had a happy baby with Gerber-quality cheeks.

When I woke up one morning soon after the birth and saw I'd missed sixteen calls, my heart dropped. I learned the baby had been admitted to the hospital after a brief resolved unexplained event (this is so common it goes by the acronym BRUE). The parents had heard a noise in the middle of the night, a grunt from the baby that was somehow different than all of the typical grunts and snorts, leading them to run and check on the baby. They found the baby altered, tense, not breathing, blue, and unresponsive. The episode lasted less than a minute, and the baby suddenly was breathing fine and his color returned to normal. The baby's condition resolved completely and on its own, but my friends were, of course, terrified.

They took their son to the emergency room and they confirmed that he had completely recovered from the episode and was well. Since his history and examination were so benign, the medical team sent him home. They suspected the episode was due to a reflux, his bedtime bottle of milk might have been irritating his upper throat and causing him to have transient difficulty breathing. They recommended some simple maneuvers to reduce reflux like holding him upright after feeds.

When I saw the family next, things were different. Tension, uncertainty, and darkness had entered their home. Because life with the new baby had been going so well, this sudden event had shocked them to the reality that the good times were no guarantee that life would continue to be easy. "What if we hadn't woken up?" they asked, with big bags under their eyes. The possibility that there was something really wrong and they might lose their baby loomed in their minds.

I can tell you that low-risk babies who have episodes like this generally have excellent outcomes. The odds are the episode was related to acid reflux and another episode may never occur. Since this event happened years ago, I can say with confidence he is now a happy, healthy third grader. But right after the episode, they were understandably terrified.

When it comes to parenting, fear is the most primal of all emotions. We know that fear activates our fight, flight, or freeze response; this triggers our adrenals to pump out stress hormones and dramatically alters our physiology. In some ways this response serves us well. It may temporarily give us the energy to do what needs to get done. However, carrying this sense of fear long-term can erode a family's well-being.

When your child has a major scare, be it a heart event, a seizure, anaphylaxis, a car accident, or a BRUE, it's only natural and expected for parents to be scared and traumatized. But often families who face less directly life-threatening challenges can feel scared too.

Joe is a six-year-old with mild cerebral palsy. His main symptom has been toe walking and his motor coordination has led to more falls. He has seen physical medicine and rehabilitation specialists, who gave him braces for his legs, and he visited orthopedic doctors who offered surgery or injections to help his tight calf muscles. He has been in physical therapy multiple times a week for as long as he can remember.

His parents may not be facing an imminent, life-threatening crisis, but their worries can be substantial. They may be concerned that his diagnosis isn't correct or that his symptoms will worsen over time. His parents may worry about inclusion and his ability to keep up with his peers, and about whether they've chosen the right providers to manage his condition. His parents might feel anxious about his pain and how it impacts his sleep. All of these worries can add up to a substantial load that is difficult to carry.

Most parents worry about making the right choices or about the uncertainty of the future. For some parents these worries can feel manageable. But for other parents the anxiety can be overwhelming. Sometimes parents try to bury the fear; shoving it aside and moving through it can feel practical, but often the anxiety will color the way you view your child and the decisions you make.

Excessive fear can lead you to distrust those around you. Parents can feel that speaking about a concern might make it come true, but this kind of magical thinking can disadvantage us from getting the support and perspective we need to manage our fear.

To approach excessive worry, I recommend prioritizing sleep, redirection, mantras, and breathing exercises—some of which I'll discuss later in this chapter. Batching worries is another technique that can help. If you set aside half an hour a week to worry, when concerns intrude on your day, you can write down a reminder to think about that later during worry time. This process can prevent worries from derailing your day and remind you that you control your thoughts.

Beware Paper Tigers

When we face stressful situations, often our brains perceive them as threats and our bodies respond with a full-out fight or flight response. We see a tiger, and we begin breathing faster, our heart beats faster, we start to sweat. These are all survival interventions designed to help us run away from that tiger.

Caregiving parents certainly face plenty of real tigers—threats to your child's well-being. But be mindful of "paper tigers." A translation of a Mandarin Chinese phrase, *zhi lao hu*, paper tigers appear threatening but are not actually able to cause harm.[4] Sometimes, we mistakenly respond to paper tigers as we might react to the real thing.

When a doctor does a physical exam of our child and finds something like a heart murmur or a developmental delay, often parents can react fearfully out of proportion with the severity of the situation. Their brain has classified this situation as a tiger, when really, it's just an area of uncertainty requiring further investigation or treatment.

If you think your anxiety may exceed the severity of what you face, pause and ask yourself: What are you actually scared of? When parents stop to parse things out, they will discover they're worried about something unlikely, like a brain tumor causing their child's headache. Or they're worried about something impractically far down the line, like their child missing out on college athletics due to a developmental delay. Sometimes, when parents just discuss the worry out loud, they can put the worry into perspective.

Anger

I once worked with a family whose teenage son had an advanced cancer. He had hidden his symptoms due to embarrassment—his scrotum was affected—and this thereby delayed his diagnosis. His mother was deeply upset with this, and felt angry with him—how could he have waited so long to speak up? I sat with her and we talked. I reminded her that it was okay to be mad at her child, even though he was really sick. She was angry because she loved him so much. And that's actually where her anger stemmed from; she was angry that her loved one had cancer, more so than she was mad that he had hidden his symptoms. And she was desperately worried about him.

When parents are given some time to calm down and reflect, it can be easier to pinpoint the source of their anger. As a parent of a child with challenges, if you feel angry, or get angry, it's likely for a good reason. Sometimes you may be frustrated with a loved one or member of your care team, but more often, that anger is diffuse and due to the unfairness of the situation. There's a lot to be angry about, but I want to assure you now: you can be a kind, loving parent and a good person and still be ferociously angry.

Anger and resentment are part of the act of caregiving, as much as we might wish they were not. More than half of family caregivers of elderly individuals report feeling anger of at least moderate intensity frequently.[5] Still, anger is as valid an emotion as any other, and most of the anger you experience as a parent and caregiver comes from an understandable place. It could be due to systemic injustice—your child may be in an unfair and difficult position and you are unable to fix it. Perhaps, as we discussed earlier, your grief about the way your life has had to change in light of your child's diagnosis has led to resentment. It's an expected and appropriate reaction. And sometimes anger, like fear, can be positive. It can spur us to address something or make a change. However, anger can also be harmful.

I find that many parents facing challenges are mad but don't have an appropriate outlet. They can't blame the child or the doctor, and they don't want to blame themselves or their co-parent. So, they just try to choke it down. It's not socially pleasant to be angry, and we don't want to upset our children by coming off as hostile.

Parents have to learn to cope with feelings of anger so they do not drive up their blood pressure or infiltrate their relationships with resentment. Pediatricians know children with disabilities are at nearly three and a half times greater risk of maltreatment, and I suspect that anger—often provoked by structural inequities—is a leading cause.[6]

I find many parents who move past the stigma of admitting they are struggling with their anger still don't seek help because they imagine no one can really help. However, there are effective ways to reduce chronic anger. In some situations, anger is a symptom of a larger problem, like burnout or depression, and treating the underlying concern with therapy or medication is the priority. Sometimes we can modify our environment in ways that reduce triggers for anger. If you find that you're routinely angry during your child's bedtime, it's likely that your reserves of patience and energy are exhausted by the end of the day. You may find that changing something can improve matters, like getting more sleep or more support, changing the routine, moving bedtime earlier, or instituting new house rules. Studies have shown that regular exercise, at least two to three days a week, decreases anger significantly.[7]

Shame

Shame is a universal emotion; considered to be a cousin of guilt, we feel shame when we feel judged by others for violating social norms—while we feel guilty for actions, we feel shamed for being ourselves. In this way, shame cuts deeper into our identity, and studies have shown that individuals who feel more shame are those who are at higher risk for depression and anxiety disorders.[8]

In my practice, I once treated a toddler experiencing poor weight gain who required feedings by nasogastric tube. This is not an uncommon intervention; the child is fed through a catheter threaded through the nose into the stomach. Once the tube is in place, it's typically well tolerated by children, but the process of insertion can be stressful—the child gags, and you need to confirm the appropriate position. Once in, a tube can stay in place for two to six weeks depending on the circumstances.

But for this toddler, every week the tube would be dislodged or have some kind of problem and need replacing. This meant more procedures and more discomfort for the child, and I couldn't understand why. Finally, the mother opened up to me. She said attending weekly church services was really important to her. Church was an important source of community, and her faith was central to her coping with her daughter's diagnosis. But Mom was struggling with the public seeing her daughter's condition and could not bring herself to bring the baby to church with a feeding tube. She felt judged and inadequate that she could not help her baby gain weight without intervention.

On top of this, the mother felt guilty for tampering with the tube weekly and hesitated to bring it up at visits. She felt that not only would her community ostracize her for using a feeding tube, but I would also judge her for not using the feeding tube as prescribed. And no, I could not entirely understand her choices. I personally felt any church community that would judge her for using a feeding tube seemed like a community ill equipped to provide the sort of support she really needed. However, stigma against illness and ableism infiltrates most institutions and I knew that Mom feeling connected to her community was important to her and her daughter's well-being. Every family has unique values and priorities, and only the family can decide what is in their child's best interest.

Once she opened up to me about her concerns, it enabled us to adjust the care plan in a way that met all the family's needs. Understanding that social inclusion, support from one's community, and self-esteem as a parent are important to the family's health and well-being, we adjusted the supplemental feeding schedule to occur mostly overnight and provided the mother with the training and supplies to remove and replace the tube more frequently around the church schedule.

Many years later, I had a family confront a similar situation. Three of their four teenage children would be undergoing confirmation at their church—a ceremony to demonstrate full commitment to their faith. For the parents, it did not seem right that their daughter would be excluded because she was unable to verbally communicate and required a wheelchair for mobility purposes. This family chose to make a different choice—requesting their child with significant disabilities be welcomed to the confirmation process within the church—something not standard previously. The church accommodated their request and subsequently more children with disabilities began to show up for services and joined the confirmation class. While this success is an inspiring example of the power of advocacy, it's worth remembering that often, particularly in very stressful times, families just want to feel comfortable and don't want to have the additional responsibility for changing the community or helping systems to evolve.

Parents struggle with shame, and we need to accept our own negative feelings about whatever challenge we face. To add to this emotional burden, parents are often required to digest other people's negative feelings. I've heard from so many parents who found the "I'm so sorry" and the "That's so terrible" reactions to their children's diagnoses upsetting. While the family members, friends, and acquaintances are usually trying to communicate empathetically, when these statements are shared, the underlying message is one of despair. When a child has a disability, many parents view it as just one part of the child's identity. But when other people feel that the child and family is defined by what they view as a *tragedy*, this view stigmatizes the family's experience.

A family may feel that there are abundant triggers for feelings of shame, and this feeling is unfortunately commonplace. Triggers crop up like potholes in the path of a family trying to do the right thing. In my practice, I've worked with mothers who wanted to quit breastfeeding because of their feelings of inadequacy when weight checks weren't going well, and I experienced this anxiety myself before starting to use supplemental formula with my daughter. Because parents facing challenges have many more interactions with medical and educational systems, there are more opportunities to feel shamed or judged. For example, individual educational plans (IEPs) are the gold standard for providing children with the physical, occupational, and speech therapy services they need, but I have had parents withdraw from services because it was just too hard to sit in a room with people talking about how a child wasn't meeting the goals.

If feelings of shame are particularly difficult for you, perhaps rethink your care plan. Is it possible to let your co-parent, babysitter, or other caregiver attend those difficult meetings or appointments in your place and report back? This distance can give you more time and privacy as you process news and results. You can also discuss your feelings with your care team and try to restructure the process into something that will work better for you. Some parents purchase their own scales or other instruments to use at home so they can feel control over the process and call me as needed. Or if you find the IEP meetings to be stressful, you can consider meeting with the providers one-on-one if your school is willing. If speaking up is challenging for you, you can ask others to do so on your behalf and on terms you feel comfortable with.

When I started prekindergarten, I was bald from cancer treatments and had an infusion port for chemotherapy. I lived two hours away from the treatment center. Yet, at my mom's request, nurses drove for hours, came to my school, and met with my class, teachers, and school nurse. They took on the work of educating my school community about my diagnosis and treatment and answered questions that might have been difficult for my family to face. Often you may find that others are willing to go out of their way like this to advocate on your behalf.

Though we live in a time of growing inclusivity, it is still not easy to be different, and we can be made to feel shame for these differences. Although it may sometimes feel unfair to be your own, or your child's, advocate, if you can speak up about your feelings you may find people who are willing to change. Ableism colors our experience, and often even well-intentioned professionals like myself can make missteps and cause feelings of discomfort. The only way to improve is through awareness. Tell me and others where we misstep—we are listening and want to do better.

I once took my son to an art class and a boy in a wheelchair entered the room with confidence. He said loudly to the art teacher, without hesitation, "These tables will not work for me. In the past I've used a table at a different height. Can you get one for me?" I wanted to bottle up his self-esteem and self-advocacy to share with my patients and other parents.

Burnout

One day, I got a fax about a case from child services requesting the medical records of one of my families. This happened almost once a month, whenever concerns for negligence or abuse were filed on one of my patients. Often these heartbreaking stories caught me off guard but weren't a surprise. I would hear about a child who had missed three appointments to have a cast removed after an orthopedic surgery, meaning a four-year-old had a cast for an extra six weeks, but I knew all the barriers they faced in getting care. In another situation, a shelter filed a complaint against a mother leaving her young children home alone to go to work. Child services has a bad reputation for splitting up families thoughtlessly—this is no longer the case. Generally, these child services cases would result in families with desperate need for support getting more resources—a free day care voucher or social work assistance with school, housing, or financial aid.

But this case surprised me. This family seemed to have it all together—stable jobs, family support, and a steady place to live. What could have happened? I called the children's mother, and the story came tumbling out. Her child had misbehaved at a hospital event and Mom, after months of dealing with insufficient sleep and excessive stress, had snapped, slapping her child in front of a dozen doctors, nurses, and social workers. As mandated reporters, her action had been flagged as abuse.

This family had two sick children. One child who needed an organ transplant and another with a congenital malformation requiring serial surgeries. Their conditions required dozens of procedures and hospital stays between the two of them. I saw the children and spoke to the mother almost every week for one reason or another—if not to address her concerns or the children's health, then to help with an insurance or school paperwork–related issue. The mother never seemed to miss a beat. She knew the meds, she kept the appointments, she knew her kids, she asked great questions. She seemed to be coping so well with all of the stress.

But as I listened to her now, she shared all of the other problems she had been dealing with on her own: the financial and emotional stress, the isolation, the relationship difficulties, and the behavioral struggles of two young kids with extra needs, including one whose medication seemed to turn her into a "monster." She was having headaches from tension and unable to sleep even when her household was calm. She was burnt-out and her irritability and difficulty coping led to the slap.

I only had one question—why didn't she say something sooner? Really it was more of a rhetorical question. Parents want to be able to do everything for their families and view caring for the children well as one of their most important jobs. Asking for help may make you feel like less of a parent. When you are in the trenches and burnt-out, you can feel hopeless—as if it is impossible that anyone could help. She wanted to avoid any judgment, including her own.

I could not fix her problems overnight, but I could connect her with a social worker to help get more financial assistance and help train some other family members to provide her with more respite. I could help reconfigure the medication and feeding schedule to try to protect her sleep more. I could talk to the specialist prescribing the medication with so many behavioral side effects to consider alternatives.

As her children's pediatrician, and after fielding so many questions regarding the kids, I wanted her to know she could come to me as well to discuss her struggles. I was part of her caregiving team too. As a pediatrician, I was here to support the children, and that also meant that I was available to support the parents. Please know that if you are struggling, there is always value in asking for help.

Are You Burnt-Out?

Psychological research indicates three main dimensions to burnout: exhaustion, detachment, and a sense of ineffectiveness. Symptoms include:

- Physical manifestations of exhaustion
  - Headaches
  - Poor sleep
  - Stomachaches

- Emotional manifestations
  - Drained of energy and creativity
  - Unable to cope with minor stressors

- Detachment or depersonalization symptoms
  - Cynicism or irritability
  - Feeling ineffective
  - Unable to concentrate
  - Feeling hopeless

If you find that you have some or all of these symptoms, please seek help to address your burnout. Many burnt-out parents lose the perspective to see that things can improve, but for many it's a question of identifying the right resource.

If you sought this book out, I can imagine it's been a difficult time for you and your family. The most common reason I see parents struggle is because the caregiving duties crowd out everything else. We're so focused on achieving our child's developmental milestones that we forget to smile, laugh, and just be present with our child. We're so frustrated by our lack of progress or the barriers to care that sap our time and energy that we disconnect from who we were prior to the challenges we encountered. Parents are often so spent from the demands, they don't have any energy left to attend to their needs, their friends, creative outlets, hobbies, recreation, and all the things that make them who they are.

If you see this happening to you, there are ways to break this cycle. As a parent, you have an essential and unavoidable job in helping your family through a challenge, but you are also at high risk for burning out.

Parental Burnout

The World Health Organization defines burnout as having three dimensions—reduced professional efficiency, exhaustion, and feelings of negativity or cynicism related to one's job. While much of the literature focuses on burnout due to work, specifically paid work outside of the home, parental burnout due to unpaid work within the home is increasingly being recognized. In 2010, a study found nearly 20 percent of parents met criteria for burnout. Looking specifically at parents of children with type 1 diabetes or inflammatory bowel disease, 36 percent—nearly twice as many—reported burnout.[9] Though my perspective is biased toward the sickest families, I feel most parents at times take on impossible loads and face excessive stress that can lead to burnout.

The pandemic brought this into focus as most parents had excessive demands on their time. Parenting and working from home while schools were closed is a good proxy for what many parents of children with chronic illness face all the time. A parent is calming the fears, reading the books, keeping the schedule, doing the laundry, serving the meals, and promoting development and learning. On top of this, caregiving parents have appointments, extra homework, additional research, equipment and medication, and school accommodations to manage. It's no wonder these parents experience higher levels of burnout.

So many parents may think, "I may be burnt-out, but it's just the way it has to be." Culturally, many parents feel to be a good parent they must tolerate excessive demands with insufficient resources. With time, I hope our society evolves to provide parents with more support (e.g., paid leave, reliable and accessible childcare). Additionally, I hope we can reduce the pressure to be a perfect and relentlessly positive parent, as these unrealistically high standards further increase perceived demands. Parental wellness—the absence of burnout—is valuable because parents' needs matter.

In my experience, most parents agree with this. When their friends suffer from burnout, they are quick to say they deserve better and support their friends in changes to improve their balance. However, the same parents often tolerate burnout themselves because of their desire to do what's best for their child. We can lose perspective easily, but burnout has unintended consequences.

Workplaces have found that burnout is associated with worsening performance. Many forward-thinking companies in the technology and banking fields have begun to give employees unlimited vacation days or require employees to take vacation for this reason. Not because of their desire to win workplace awards, but because they know that employees who are rested are more productive. Similarly, burnt-out parents can see how their exhaustion can lead to reduced efficiency as they are unable to focus or complete the necessary tasks due to fatigue.

With parenting, burnout's impact on families has the potential to be more toxic than what we observe in the workplace. Imagine how feelings of detachment might impair our close connections with our family and our support system. Instinctively we know that when we feel hopeful, optimistic, or positive about our future, we're more likely to set higher goals and work more energetically toward positive outcomes.

Harriet was a three-year-old girl who had survived prematurity and congenital heart disease. She had not yet walked or learned to talk, but we had reasons to be optimistic about her future acquisition of these skills given her recent improvements—her heart was now fixed and her strength and stamina to work toward gaining new skills improved. Her family had been through a terrible time—dozens of hospitalizations, multiple near-death experiences, and she had been suspected to have had a stroke more than once. Feeling overwhelmed by all the intrusions on their time, her family decided to opt out of all of her therapies. This was not a break—they wanted to be done.

When I asked them why and tried to see things from their perspective, I learned that in some ways they had given up on her. In the past, they had been through cycles of having hope only to see a setback occur. Their love for her was unconditional, and they didn't expect that she would learn more skills. Their acceptance of the status quo was a coping mechanism, but this learned negativity acquired from recurrent trauma was leading them to close off doors to interventions that might help. Even if the goals of therapy were not to acquire these milestones, therapy still could benefit her by preventing complications from her disability, like pain. We ended up negotiating a break with minimal therapies. Once the parents saw her stable and improving, we made plans for her to go to school and get all the services she needed.

While cynicism can be a way to protect ourselves from further disappointments, research has shown it to be a health hazard.[10] While the research on this topic for now consists mostly of small observational studies, you can imagine that optimistic perspectives would open doors to opportunities or help families find more resources and more support. Theoretically, this parental optimism could enable children to achieve better outcomes. Parental burnout and the related hopelessness and exhaustion would instead reduce a parent's ability to optimally care for their children.

How to Break the Burnout Cycle

It feels trite to encourage self-care to parents who already have so much on their plate—because the demands on you are fixed due to your child's needs, and because of the way the health and educational systems are constructed. Pooja Lakshmin, a psychiatrist and women's mental health advocate, may have put it best when she spoke of stress loads reflecting societal betrayal, not personal burnout.[11] Burnout in many ways is not a problem you can fix as a parent. Caregiver burnout is a systemic problem. Our society undervalues the work of caregivers and assumes that parents should handle all caregiving on their own without outside help. But even when systemic change seems unlikely in the short-term, it still helps for us to find ways we can promote our coping and prioritize well-being.

Prioritizing Your Own Wellness

Parents are often the best advocates for their children's health care. But as we've discussed, there is only so much time, so much energy, and so many resources. When families devote it all to the children, sometimes parents end up relatively neglected.

However, your needs matter, especially basic needs like sleep, exercise, and regular meals. If you don't attend to these basic needs, you risk compromising your health and happiness. You may be more irritable or have worse judgment. Anxiety will be heightened. In the short-term, we feel like we can power through, but in the longer term the cost of neglecting these basic needs will become more significant and your health may be compromised.

You are really too important to your family to be neglected.

It's essential that you're in the best mental and emotional state you can be. Many have heard the caregiving analogy that parents need to put on their own oxygen mask first, so to speak, on airplanes and in life. This advice may lead some of you to roll your eyes, but it's also a reality that a caregiver who is sleeping, eating regular meals, and keeping an active social life will be better prepared to show up for their child when it matters.

In addition to these basic needs, increasing positive emotions in your life helps to promote resilience. Creative outlets like dance, art, poetry, photography, or crafting can reduce feelings of burnout and promote feelings of self-efficacy. Connecting with people or activities you love can also help tip the balance toward positive feelings crowding out the negative. Helping others—such as advocating and mentoring other families in your position—can make you feel good and help you to find meaning. Gratitude—savoring these positive experiences—can further magnify the perception of positivity in your life.

When you are dealing with a system that doesn't seem to work for you and your family, you need to remember that you can advocate for your own needs. Parents have a tendency to martyr themselves for their children. But despite societal messaging to the contrary, it doesn't make you a less loving or considerate parent if you spend time and energy prioritizing yourself. In fact, it may make you a better parent.

Set and Defend Your Limits

One essential way to make time and space and reclaim energy for yourself as a parent is to set limits. You are allowed to say, "No," "That won't work," or, "It's too much." You can say no to your child even if it's something they really want. You can say no to something the school asks you to do. You can say no to something your doctor recommends. If ever a request doesn't make sense to you or feels excessive, you have rights. No one knows your family like you do and you may know that sometimes *not* doing more may be what's in your best interest.

Perhaps your child is having speech difficulties and you've been referred for a hearing test and to start therapy. That's all fine, but you are going to have a new baby any day and have limited bandwidth for extra issues. For some children, like a child who is having severe tantrums and significantly stalled speech development, having a timely hearing test and starting the process sooner may be essential. If your two-year-old isn't speaking and you learn there is a fixable cause of hearing loss, addressing it promptly will help promote language development and reduce your family stress level, even amidst the busyness of planning for birth.

But in other situations, like a five-year-old with a slight speech impairment, delaying starting therapy for six months may be no big deal if it will be easier for you logistically at that time. This goes back to the priorities and big picture we discussed earlier in Chapter 2. While these examples are relatively obvious, most situations fall somewhere in the middle, and often I find the most important part of my discussions with parents is the part where I clarify how the issues fit in the context of the rest of their lives.

There can be perceived power imbalances between health care and educational practitioners and parents, such that caregiving parents may hesitate to question recommended care. You don't want to upset the principal or teachers running the Individualized Education Program meeting, because you need them to help your child. If the doctor is recommending something, you feel it must be important, and you worry that if you question the plan, you may somehow offend them. While these individuals bring experience and knowledge to approaching these decisions, ultimately, as the parent, you know your family and your child best. Professionals in these fields supporting families facing challenges should value your perspective and respect your authority as the decision maker.

Delegate

Thoughtfully doing less may be the most effective way to reduce your stress level. But often you may feel you can't. If you are feeling overwhelmed by all you have to do, delegation is something to explore; but to be clear, delegation is not a simple solution—it comes with logistic, financial, and emotional costs.

However, in many situations, we imagine the barriers to be larger and more troubling than they are in reality. Some things only a parent can do—making medical decisions, helping a child in extreme distress, and leading a family. But other people can be trained to do many of the day-to-day tasks of a parent with training and effort—meal prep, household management, medication administration, or child transportation. Investing the time and energy into setting up a new workflow can pay off. Sometimes we underestimate how others can step in for us when needed. While a babysitter, relative, or neighbor may not supervise meals or bedtime in the same way you do, if they are doing a fine job and your child is cared for, it should be enough. Essentially, the cost of an imperfect solution may still justify the benefit of a break. Some children are particularly fragile or have very specialized caregiving needs, and you may be especially intimidated to train a babysitter, but in these situations do not forget that you can ask for help from professionals involved with your child to ensure the child's safety.

We are especially slow to delegate cognitive labor, simply because we care about our children more than anyone else and we can't imagine that anyone else could be trusted to anticipate and monitor complex situations. But when responsibilities are clearly delineated, often others can be trained to be conscientious.

If your child's challenge is short-term in nature, you may feel as if you can take on all of the added responsibilities and bulldoze your way through it for a few months. However, stop to consider whether this is really what's best for your family. Many parents may see that childhood is one challenge after another, particularly if you have multiple children.

If you do take it on by yourself, you may be more likely to experience burnout and be less happy and less effective. Finding a way to share the challenge with your co-parent or support system may make it more manageable for you *and* may result in improving the big picture plan.

If your child's challenge is expected to be long-term, burnout—both for you and your child—is something to be mindful of. It's easy to fall into routines that do not promote our well-being; having limits, adjusting your limits over time, delegating, prioritizing yourself, and taking breaks can help you prevent getting to that burnt-out state.

If you do feel burnt-out, know that it's possible to work your way out of it. Small changes can add up to big relief over time, and even when it's not immediately evident how to make things better, recognizing how you feel is the first step to making changes. Big picture, spending the energy to get yourself to a better place will help you and your family.

We've just reviewed all the difficult feelings that parents can face when their child has a challenge. In the next section we'll talk about what to do about it and review ways to feel better.

- If the description of burnout resonates with what you are experiencing, what can you do to change your situation?
- Be honest and reflect on the last few weeks: Have you taken care of yourself?
- Think about your limits. Is there anything you could say no to, to preserve your energy?
- Pick one task that you would really like to delegate and consider: What's stopping you?
- If you aren't burnt-out, is your current arrangement sustainable?

What to Do to Feel Better

We started this chapter exploring many of the difficult emotions parents feel—sadness and grief, guilt, fear and anxiety, anger, shame and burnout. Depending on your specific situation, you may relate to a lot of these uncomfortable feelings or only a few. One reason it can be so difficult to have negative feelings about your parenting journey is the mismatch between what you expected and what you face. Many of us expect parenthood to be all "unicorns and rainbows," and the hard part is not expected or welcome. This can be particularly challenging for parents who find their situation is harder or more complex than a typical parenting journey.

As you reflect on which of these feelings you are experiencing or have experienced in the past, remember: parenting isn't always easy or fun. Even when things are going well, you may not love every minute—and you don't have to. When your child faces a challenge, you will experience even more negative feelings. It doesn't mean that you are a bad parent if the negative emotions outweigh the positive emotions sometimes. You can dislike some parts of parenting but still love your child.

Not only is it okay to give yourself permission to find help, but in the long run finding ways to release these emotions may also help your health and your family relationships. When I talk to parents about these feelings, I hear concerns like these:

- "The feeling is so big it feels like it may overwhelm me."
- "The feeling is so selfish that I feel ashamed of it."
- "Sometimes just acknowledging its existence feels like a betrayal."

Our negative thoughts and feelings are more overwhelming when they are kept to ourselves. When you can open up about them, you can take the first steps to making them feel more manageable and working through them. Remember as you face these difficult feelings that you aren't alone.

Many parents shy away from opening up with themselves or their support system about their negative feelings. We worry that others will judge us or that we're the only ones who have these types of feelings. Beyond that, being a caregiver to a child with a challenge can be inherently isolating and the loneliness can be its own hardship to process.

When life takes you down a different path, there are fewer people who can understand what you're going through. Our society has historically marginalized people with mental health concerns, chronic illness, or learning disabilities. Parents worry that a label or a diagnosis may lead to exclusion or uncomfortable questions and in response they often turn inward. But, like most things in life, it's unlikely we are the only ones who feel a certain way or are experiencing this set of challenges.

Your child's challenge will most certainly have an impact on you, and only you can understand the severity of that impact and the type of support you need. Having professional help in confronting some of the hard feelings associated with parenting is never a bad idea, but it becomes particularly essential when the negative feelings begin to crowd out the positive feelings.

Caregiving stress that exceeds and overwhelms a parent's capacity to cope can lead to clinical depression or anxiety. Studies have shown that considerable percentages of parents of children who face challenges, like a car accident or cancer, experience symptoms consistent with post-traumatic stress disorder.

If you are currently feeling overwhelmed by the negative feelings you face, you should know that there are treatments and solutions that can help. Some people who are struggling will need the help of a doctor or mental health provider who can provide therapy, medication, or a combination approach. Evidence-based therapy such as cognitive behavioral therapy (CBT) has emerged as the gold standard for many behavioral health conditions.[12] CBT involves learning to recognize distorted thinking processes, developing problem-solving skills, and changing behavior patterns. Many find that these interventions yield significant benefits in as few as six to eight sessions.[13] Other people find that long-term therapy is needed to help them with significant anxiety or depression.

If you aren't sure if therapy is right for you, please err on the side of speaking with a trained professional. By far the most common reason I hear parents hesitate to seek care is that they don't have time. But for something so important, that will impact your relationships and day-to-day well-being, you may have to make time. Be mindful that it can take time to find the right professional and to get treatment started. Taking concrete steps to obtain help can work well in parallel with trying some new coping skills discussed in this book. In the resource list, I've included several online options for seeking mental health care as well as some options for finding it at a reduced-fee scale. If your self-help efforts work, you could always cancel an appointment or discuss seeing your provider less frequently, but don't underestimate the benefit of having an expert on mental health support give you tailored advice, direct you toward specific local resources, and monitor your response to treatment over time.

In the next section, we'll dive into some of the coping skills that parents can use. Even if you are mostly in a healthy frame of mind, these skills are wonderful tools to keep you there. These tools can also help you model resilience for your children and family members.

Coping Toolbox

Parents facing a child's challenge are typically in a high-stakes, high-stress situation. The uncertainty and the lack of control worsen the frustration for many parents. Earlier, we touched on how we all have our strengths and weaknesses, and that we all have a personal habitual response to stress. Now I'd like to discuss skills we can learn to improve our coping abilities. Even if these don't feel natural, these tools can expand and improve your capacity to cope.

Awareness

Our response to stress consists mostly of how we feel, rather than what we think or say. When aggravated, our pulse quickens and we begin to sweat. We transition to feeling threatened, and our responses become more aggressive or defensive. We might say we are "fine," but our tone and body language show otherwise. If we want to change that response pattern to one that is more positive or constructive, it's essential to first notice that physiological transition to aggravation.

We know that children in midtantrum can't be reasoned with. Similarly, when we are in a dysregulated, stressed state, we can't respond with intention. Staying in tune with your body's reaction is essential, yet remarkably easy to forget. Some people are tuned in to their stress level, but others, like myself, are not. When I feel overwhelmed, I have to make a concerted effort to keep my shoulders from creeping up toward my ears and I have to consciously avoid my default "bulldozer" mode from taking over.

Some parents have described this stressed state to me as their "seeing red." Others feel as if they are shutting down, like a turtle pulling into their shell. Identifying and allowing yourself to feel this way is the first step to changing it, and sometimes we can help ourselves get to a better spot.

Positive Self-Talk

We all have an inner monologue as we go about our day-to-day. When something isn't going our way, we might express things like:

> "I just can't get this right."
> "These people are impossible."
> "I am messing up my kid."
> "I will never be as good a parent as..."
> "This will never end."

These sorts of statements cast a parent as incapable, a victim, a hazard, and trapped. But in addition to making a parent feel worse about the situation, they reinforce the idea that things are fixed the way they are and hopeless. When things are hard, it would be inauthentic and Pollyannaish to sugarcoat it excessively. But growth mindsets have been trending for a reason—it's a free, evidence-based way to improve your outlook.

If you catch yourself saying these negative statements to yourself, see if you can change them into more constructive statements or questions.

Negative Statements	Constructive Statements
"I just can't get this right."	"I am struggling with this; how can I get help?"
"These people are impossible."	"What could I do to work this system differently?"
"I am messing up my kid."	"I am doing the best I can, but I'm not happy with the result yet."
"I will never be as good a parent as..."	"He seems to do a great job at this part of parenting; what could I learn from him?"
"This will never end."	"What can I change to make this more sustainable?"

The combination of recognizing your feelings and exercising self-compassion has been studied and suggested as an intervention to promote parental coping.[14] The purpose of this is to learn how to acknowledge negative feelings. When these feelings go unacknowledged, they can incite a negative feedback loop of poor self-talk and worsening coping.

Guided Imagery

Many people hear the term "guided imagery" and roll their eyes. However, guided imagery is a well-established stress-management technique, and there is a ton of evidence showing that it helps.

Our brains are incredibly powerful, and when we can train ourselves to imagine ourselves in nature or another relaxing restorative place, the results can be impressive. One study showed a nearly 25 percent reduction in anxiety with one ten-minute visualization session.[15] Research suggests that imagining a relaxing, restorative place is actually more effective than spending time there—likely because of the practical issues that preclude enjoyment in the moment. When you imagine a peaceful place, you don't have to deal with the sun feeling too hot or the sand irritating your skin.

Guided imagery certainly helps with stress, anxiety, and depression, but has also been investigated to reduce pain and blood pressure and enhance recovery. If you want to try guided imagery, take a moment somewhere comfortable to imagine a place and time when you were truly happy, or a moment when you were surrounded by natural beauty that took your breath away. Then remember the sounds, smells, sights, and textures you encountered.

If you don't have time to dedicate toward focused meditation, you may still find that even brief interventions can be helpful. When you "see red" and feel angry, you can imagine calm blue waves. If you notice that your arms are closed and you are withdrawing, you can imagine a turtle pulling into its shell, take a deep breath, and relax your posture. If you feel like you are caught in a downpour, you can imagine a duck with waterproof feathers shaking off the excess water. These images may not resonate with everyone, but they can be a nonverbal way to guide you into relaxation when you are facing stress.

When we are protecting our child's well-being, we have a tendency to focus on all the things that can go wrong. Sometimes guided imagery can be used to imagine things going well, and in doing so foster creative problem-solving and hope. Athletes often imagine positive outcomes before a competition begins, and studies show that this does improve performance.[16]

Meditations, Mantras, and Breathing Exercises

Busy people sometimes feel meditation is a luxury—something out of reach for most of us. When I spoke with parents about how they made it through difficult times, they often referenced moments of peace. Moments when they could relax or forget about their stress and focus on something else. They might consider their weekly favorite TV show or a piece of chocolate a "treat," but it's important for all parents to slow down and take a moment for themselves from time to time. Some people can find absorption in self-care tasks, like showering or washing the dishes. When your hands are busy, you are unable to multitask and your mind may have room to wander. Others may find moving meditation useful; they may take a walk or a run and attempt to breathe in the moment.

Finding a phrase that resonates with your tough emotions can help you feel better too. The magic of a short phrase is that once it becomes a habit, it can provide some peaceful continuity to your day. Parents have found different mantras to be helpful:

- "I'm doing the best I can."
- "Tomorrow is a new day."
- "Progress, not perfection."
- "I can only control myself."
- "I am the perfect parent for my child."
- "I am not alone."
- "Calm is contagious."

Some believe that most relaxation and coping techniques work because of how they affect one's breathing. When we slow our respirations, we activate our parasympathetic nervous system, enhancing our feelings of emotional control and psychological well-being.[17] I often teach children box breathing:

1. Place your hand on your stomach so you can feel the in and out of breathing with your hand.
2. Breathe in for a count of four.
3. Hold it for a count of four.
4. Breathe out for a count of four.
5. Hold it for a count of four.

Repeating these steps even a few times will aid in relaxation.

Finding Outlets for Humor

Sometimes I imagine trying to cope as analogous to trying to use a dish-cloth to wipe up spills. The cloth works well for a while, absorbing stains left and right, but eventually needs to be thrown in the washing machine and reset for more work ahead. For us, how do we reset, when we know more stress and frustration will come again and again?

Perhaps you have a hobby—when you are feeling angry, smashing a tennis ball or running at a sprint can release a ton of tension in a relatively productive way. Journaling or connecting with other people provide other avenues to unload. But one of my favorite outlets is humor.

Joseph, an eleven-year-old boy, had always had poor endurance. He never wanted to walk, run, or bike—he would only sit around and do sedentary activities. He vigorously protested during gym class, and he got into explosive fights with his family when they required him to participate in activities like walking to the grocery store.

He was seen by multiple doctors who saw nothing wrong with him. He began therapy because of how much discord this caused in his family life. Then he screened positive for tuberculosis and the protocol required an X-ray image of his chest. He had no outward signs of tuberculosis, but his heart was nearly four times the normal size for his age. He had a rare heart defect and needed an immediate heart transplant.

I supported the family through the process of preparing for a heart transplant—and they kept *laughing* and *laughing* about it. All these years of frustration and fighting with him, thinking he had a difficult temperament or their parenting was insufficient, and now learning there was a real, tangible, fixable reason for it.

They laughed during the blood draw, they laughed during the EKG. They laughed telling me the story, nearly to the point of tears. When I asked the mom about it, she said, "Well, I guess I could either laugh at how ridiculous and unlikely and surprising this all is, or I could cry about how terrible it is that we didn't know this years ago. Somehow laughing feels better."

This chapter may have touched on some difficult topics, but in many ways, it's the most important in the book. The isolation parents face in these situations comes at a time when parents are also awash in stress and emotional fallout. I want you to know that these big, hard feelings are expected and normal and you are not alone.

There is a Buddhist teaching called the "second arrow." When something bad happens and we are hit by an arrow, it hurts. But sometimes in reaction to the first arrow, we blame ourselves. We feel guilty or ashamed that we didn't dodge it; we feel devalued because we failed and will now require help from others. Our anger and frustration turn inward. This second attack is called the "second arrow," and the goal of this discussion has been to help us recognize it. The first arrow you're facing, your child's challenge, you may have little control over. But you can control your response to it, potentially dodging the impact of the second arrow.

There is no such thing as a bad feeling; feelings just exist. You are not the only parent who is coping with difficult feelings. Once you acknowledge and accept these feelings, you can make a plan for your own well-being. You can learn to cope, you can gain new skills, you can envision a better future for yourself and your family.

Sometimes when we learn about our own feelings and coping, it can help us support other members of the family too—including our children who are at the center of all this, after all. In the next chapter, we'll talk about when your child resists treatment. We are mindful that the resistance is sometimes the tip of the iceberg, and what drives it can be our children coping with all of the difficult feelings we've discussed in this chapter too. We'll share strategies to support them and help them get the care they need.

Before moving on from this chapter:

- Reflect on how you feel now and how you've felt in the past.
- What feelings are hardest for you to cope with?
- Are your difficult feelings in proportion to the stress you face?
- Do you need more mental health support than a book can provide?
- What coping skills work best for you? Are there new ones you would consider trying?

CHAPTER 10

Understanding Your Child's Resistance

My dear friend's daughter Emily has epilepsy. It all began when she was a fifth grader and she had a few incidents where she fell over unexpectedly. Was she just clumsy? Was she distracted? The mother began to get concerned about these episodes, though she hadn't witnessed one yet. And around that time, her school called to say that she had fallen and had a seizure. All of her friends had seen her in distress with her arms and legs shaking. The school staff called 911, and at the hospital she was examined and diagnosed with epilepsy. The epilepsy likely explained the unexpected falls as well. She was started on twice-daily medication, which controlled her seizures without many side effects.

One of the hardest parts of Emily's diagnosis was the struggle to get her to take her medication. She was generally a thoughtful, kind girl and a bright, conscientious student, but she simply hated taking the medication. Twice daily, the parents struggled to get her to take it. They did not particularly like giving her medication, but they knew it was important to prevent another seizure. They just wanted her to take it and spare them all the drama, and they were exhausted. So, they asked for help.

While medication seems like an easy solution, like any other behavior change, it can be a challenge. If you've ever had to take medication regularly, you may understand that it's not as easy as it sounds. First you have to have the medication refilled and available when you need to take it, even if you're traveling or out of your routine. Then you must remember to take the medication following the instructions such as on an empty stomach or on a specific schedule. And when it's a daily medication, this burden can weigh on you.

For children, there are even more barriers. Primarily, they don't understand why they have to take the medication. Medications are unpalatable and uncomfortable. For Emily, she just did not want to do it. She would experience behavioral meltdowns, kicking and screaming like a toddler instead of the ten-year-old she was. She would spit and cry. She would hide the medication or lie and tell one parent the other had already given it to her.

When parents bring this up during a visit, I generally have very little time to dig deep. I recommend things like trying tablets instead of liquid if appropriate or tying the medication to part of the regular daily routine like brushing teeth. I have a handful of techniques I recommend for squirmy toddlers. These practical techniques may help some families, but as I spoke to my friend about their situation, I realized these workarounds were unlikely to be successful with a bright tween.

In this chapter, we'll talk about what to do when you're really hitting a wall in your efforts to help your child face their challenge. It may not be that medications are your issue; it could be taking care of a feeding tube site or getting a child to participate productively in therapy. What all of these situations share is that generally these tasks are left to the caregiver to handle, and a lot of caregivers have to learn on their own what will work in practice for their child.

The first thing I'd encourage is to reframe the problem. Emily's mother had said, "I just can't get her to take the medication." While this may feel true, viewing the problem as the parent's problem is incorrect. The child is having trouble taking the medication.

This may seem like a silly distinction, but if we view this as the parent's problem, in some ways it assigns culpability and guilt. If *you* can't get your child to take the medication, *you* must be doing something wrong, which is not the case. It could be that most children would comply with requests like the ones you are making to your child.

When we recenter our understanding of the resistance as the *child's* problem, we remember that the responsibility and ultimate solution has to be centered around the child. If we think of it as the parent's problem, we will ask questions like: When are you giving it? Where are you storing it? What script do you use to ask the child? But when it's the child's problem, we'll ask different questions, like: Why does the child not want to take it? Is it the taste or the temperature? Is it the time of day? Is it the side effects? What changes could make it easier?

Of course, sometimes it may be a struggle for both parent and child. Emily's mother may be feeling ambivalent about giving her medication and being less firm. Children can be incredibly perceptive and pick up on this hesitancy, becoming more hesitant themselves. It's possible that the caregiver could address their hard feelings or do more research to gain skills for medication administration or increase confidence in the plan and this could improve matters. But often resistance stems from the child, and in this chapter, we will focus on exploring the source of the child's resistance.

As you work to understand your child's resistance, it's important to ground your understanding in the reality of your child's developmental stage and whether what you are experiencing is typical and expected. Often caregiving parents are put into unfamiliar situations. While there are dozens of books about confronting a toddler's resistance to getting dressed or potty training, there's little out there about confronting resistance to wearing glasses, to proper wound care, to showing up at therapy, or any of the many things you may be facing.

When Your Child Puts Their Foot Down

When your child vigorously opposes a necessary activity, the first step is to understand why. Ask yourself the following questions:

- Is the expectation that my child tolerates this realistic and developmentally appropriate?

- Does this seem like it will pass quickly or does this require rethinking the plan?
- Is my child in a less receptive frame of mind? I often consider the acronym HALTS—Hungry, Angry, Lonely, Tired, or Sick (including in pain).

These straightforward questions may lead you to better understand the source of the resistance. Tackling the source can be more effective than scripts or packaging around the delivery of the treatment. Sometimes children have developmental or sensory needs such that interventions that might work for other children do not fit their needs. Even seasoned educators and physicians can't always know what kids can handle until they try. If your gut as a parent says your child cannot be expected to handle this, sometimes you may be right, and you may need help revising the plan.

Motivational Interviewing

For children and adults who are able to engage in conversation, motivational interviewing is an evidence-based technique to help prompt behavior change. At its very core, it relies on respect for the individual. Rather than saying, "You have to; just do it." Motivational interviewing would have us say, "How is it going for you having epilepsy and needing to take your medication every day?" And then you have to listen, with an open mind, to their responses.

The emotional burden this technique places on the parent should not be underestimated, because what the child says in response may be difficult to hear. The parent will instinctively want to "fix" matters, and they may not be able to, despite listening to their child's concerns. The child may be angry and feel like it's unfair. The child may feel ashamed and feel like the medication makes her feel worse. The child may be feeling all the difficult feelings we discussed earlier in the book, and they may have less capacity to cope than an adult. But hopefully, by providing a space for the child to discuss these feelings, we can help the child.

Once you have listened, then you can continue to ask open-ended questions: "Do you understand why you need the medication? Do you understand what might happen if you don't take it? What do you think we could do to make this easier for you?" By actively listening and reflecting back to the child affirmations and summaries, you can further your connection with the child and work to establish a dynamic of shared decision-making.

As you move them closer to changing their behavior, you might point out discrepancies—such as, "I heard you say you don't want to have another seizure and you want to prevent that, but when you skip the medication a few times a week you increase the risk of seizure." When you are trying to cultivate an older kid's self-management skills, it is important to resist the urge to tell them what to do and fix the problem. Unintentionally, you can lead children to dig in their heels and worsen resistance. By listening with empathy and understanding their motivation, you can empower the child to take more responsibility and control over their care and to feel proud for doing so in a way congruent with their values.

For Emily, taking the seizure medication was a twice-daily reminder that she was different, that she was at risk for another seizure, and that her friends had seen her in a vulnerable moment. She knew why she needed the medicine, but taking it triggered hard feelings, which led her to avoid the medicine. With all this information, we could together make a better plan leaning on her strengths (understanding and acceptance of the need to take medication) to find a way to make the action of taking the medication less sad. Instead of tying the medication to a time of day that was already a little stressful, like leaving to go to school or at bedtime, we could try having her take it a different time of day along with doing something fun or a little treat. By engaging her as a thought partner in picking the new plan, we set her up to feel agency and control over the choices made and increase her likelihood of success. Engaging in this type of dialogue with your child also helps you connect with them—they feel you understand where they are coming from, and you learn important information about school dynamics.

When Your Child Can't or Won't Tell You the Problem

I once took care of a six-year-old girl named Maria who had been born extremely preterm. Because she spent nearly the first six months of her life with a tube down her throat helping her breathe, she had a narrowing of her airway that required a permanent breathing tube—a tracheostomy. We hoped that as she grew, and with repeated procedures to open up her airway, she would be able to safely live without the breathing tube, but for now it was necessary. Because of the breathing tube and some developmental delays related to prematurity, Maria had difficulty expressing herself and pretty intense tantrums when she got upset.

For this family, her behavioral challenges came to a head when it was time to clean and care for the tracheostomy tube twice a day. Maria did not like it—it was uncomfortable and required her to sit still. She would thrash around, hitting Mom or sometimes hitting herself. She would at times get so agitated she would throw up. The care should only take a minute, but for them it was a process that took at least half an hour and left them both feeling exhausted.

Because Maria was unable to engage with us about how to change the plan due to her limited communication skills, Mom and I were left grasping for ways to make it better. If you find yourself in this situation, with children too young to engage in motivational interviewing who are refusing to participate in their own care, close observation and analysis of the situation can help.

In Maria's situation, we found the answer from talking with her school nurse. Because she was at school nearly eight hours, on school days she had her tracheostomy care at school. When Mom called to see how this was going, she was surprised to learn that it was a nonissue— Maria sailed through it without complaint. Mom went and observed the process—learning ways to set up the required materials before engaging Maria. The nurse explained how at the beginning of the school year she had practiced with Maria, numbering and explaining each step of the process so she knew what was coming. Since the nurse already knew Maria, she was able to coach Mom toward making the process better, though it wasn't easy. The nurse taught Mom to think about the following:

- Adding structure to the process—setting out the materials, telling Maria, and being consistent.
- Reconsidering the time of day—tracheostomy care in the evening was going to be harder for Maria because by that time in the day she was tired with less patience. Eventually Mom began doing it in the morning.
- Distraction—the nurse had a disco ball that she used with music to distract Maria from what was happening on her neck. She and Mom brainstormed about what would work best to distract Maria at home.
- Rewards—at school Maria was incentivized to finish the care quickly to return to free play time in her classroom. Mom began saving a special toy for Maria to play with after finishing at home.

One mistake parents sometimes make is rushing. Particularly with young children, everything can take extra time. Patience with yourself and your child is often required. Often it takes multiple trials of different techniques and time to adjust to new routines.

Ask for Help

Just as Maria's mom did, I would encourage parents not to hesitate to ask for help. Too often the medical system discourages follow-up questions or challenges to the initial plan, but the plan is only a good plan if it works for your family and respects the needs of the people involved. Allowing your child to go back and directly discuss the plan with the doctor will allow them to hear the same information from another credentialed voice. Maybe the plan can be adjusted; for example, if a child with strep throat really puts up a huge fight taking daily antibiotics orally, an injection can be given instead. The very act of revisiting the plan with the doctor can also be therapeutic—allowing the child to air their frustrations and complaints and feel heard.

Sometimes nurses; educators; physical, occupational, and speech therapists; or other parents may have really practical suggestions for how to help children follow through with a plan of care, so being open with others on your care team can help you to find solutions. Some examples:

- A behavioral plan like a sticker chart with a reward at the end—notably, not just for little kids, big kids can rally around this when it resonates with their goals too.
- Finding a more comfortable position to give a child medication or allowing a child to give themselves the medication (or perform their own finger stick or wound care with instruction and supervision).
- Making physical therapy exercises into a fun or social game.

While it can feel disorienting and new when you are supporting your child in facing a challenge, remember that the skills you have used to help your child tolerate a diaper change, a bath, or sunscreen, and the techniques you used to corral their cooperation with trimming nails, wearing gloves, or going to the dentist, may help. Even if those skills don't directly translate, recalling what's worked in the past may help you brainstorm ideas for what to try, leaning into your specific family's strengths and preferences.

Is Resistance Something More?

When children are struggling, addressing the root cause will be the most efficient way forward. I encourage parents to think about where the resistance is coming from, particularly if it changes abruptly. Treatment resistance can be a sign of a deeper emotional reaction to a child's situation—anxiety, burnout, depression, or trauma.

Is Your Child Worried or Anxious?

Fear, uncertainty, and lack of control often lead children to withdraw, refuse, and act out. Children often worry for valid reasons such as to avoid pain. For most children, anticipating can be worse than actual medical treatments. Medical play can help decrease fear and uncertainty—modeling how you take pretend medication, pretending to change a bandage on a stuffed animal, or giving make-believe shots to family members. Relaxation and breathing exercises can help a child tolerate the stress of an unwanted treatment. Practice sessions where you go through the motions and just take candy or juice instead of medication can help a child adjust to uncomfortable feelings. Offering choices and ways to give your child the perception of control can help too.

Routines can decrease worries by enhancing feelings of safety—the child knows what's coming. With time and repetition, children adjust to new activities and cope with fear.

However, sometimes worries begin to interfere with necessary care and worries interfere with multiple parts of the day. Worries that are leading to harm or impairment can be a sign of an underlying anxiety disorder. Anxiety is the most common child-onset psychiatric diagnosis and can present subtly in children, but there are treatments available, so it's important to recognize.

In addition to feeling worried, children with anxiety often have a few of the following symptoms.[1]

- Restlessness
- Easy to fatigue
- Difficulty concentrating
- Irritability

- Muscle tension
- Sleep disturbance
- Stomachaches or headaches

If your child seems to have anxiety, please discuss treatment options with your pediatrician.

Is Your Child Burnt-Out?

In the last chapter, I spoke about parental burnout, but it's so important to realize children are at risk for burnout as well. When your child is really putting their foot down regarding their treatment, being burnt-out is one possibility. Burnout was originally imagined as an occupational hazard, but for children, school and medical care are perceived as obligations like work demands. Children who feel exhausted, detached, or cynical about their treatment may be burnt-out.

I've seen children burnt-out from intensive interventions and from more moderate interventions that last a long time. A delightful patient of mine, a twelve-year-old named Alejandro, had difficulty with speech. He had a tongue-tie release, a surgery on his jaw, a palate expander, and years of speech therapy as often as three times a week. He was a diligent child who worked so hard on the issue, and his improvement was substantial. But before he graduated from speech therapy, his progress stalled.

He wasn't complaining excessively, but he was feeling hopeless about ever speaking clearly. He was more sensitive to the examinations of his mouth. He was no longer joking around with his speech therapist or really participating enthusiastically as he had before. And it was understandable. He had been through so much.

Notably, other areas of his life were unaffected. He really enjoyed playing with his friends and he was sleeping and eating well. He could joke with his family and his grades were good. He was crankier than normal, but mostly around the time of day he had his therapy appointments or whenever his parents reminded him to practice.

His mother and therapist were hesitant to pull back, as he was getting closer and closer to reaching their goals. But we ended up giving him a summer off. No appointments, no therapy. Just being a kid and having fun. And when he came back to therapy in the fall, the mischievous sparkle in his eye returned and he was able to engage again. Clearly, all Alejandro needed was a break.

When a Break Isn't Possible

Though even a short break can make a big difference, sometimes time away from a challenge isn't possible. When a child is burnt-out, they can benefit from all the things we discussed for parents in the prior chapter. When children are burnt-out:

- Focus on wellness staples like adequate sleep, exercise, and other coping skills.
- Be certain they spend time connecting with loved ones.
- During quality time, take a break from talking about the challenge, practicing skills, or any "work," and enjoy each other's company.
- Increase positive feelings like gratitude, belonging, and joy.
- Use favorite activities to distract them from tough times.
- Help ensure they have access to play and creative outlets.

All these experiences can help buffer children against the chronic stress they may face.

Could Your Child Be Depressed?

Even with the most thoughtful parenting, facing a challenge can be really hard for a child—so, frustrations and negative feelings are to be expected. Allowing your child safe outlets for these feelings is essential. Many caregiving parents find tolerating their child's big feelings to be a heavy weight, and sometimes children are less willing to share their big feelings with their parents—utilizing grandparents, school counselors, or therapists to help listen can be helpful for both parent and child.

However, and as much as we might want to deny it, we must also consider the possibility that your child is experiencing depression. We know that children as young as three can be diagnosed with depression and that it's more common in children with chronic illness.[2] One of the trickiest things about recognizing pediatric depression is that children frequently lack the cognitive and emotional sophistication to organize their emotional experiences. While adults might express feeling sad, children sometimes express themselves as more irritable than sad. Depressed children may feel annoyed, grouchy, or bothered by everyone. Their behavior may be argumentative, and they may seek fights.

Other symptoms of depression include the following:[3]

- Diminished interest or pleasure
- Change in appetite or weight
- Sleep disturbances
- Feeling notably restless or slow
- Fatigue or lack of energy
- Feelings of worthlessness or guilt
- Impaired concentration
- Suicidal thoughts or intentions

While exhaustion and negativity can be prominent symptoms of both burnout and depression, depression is unlikely to improve with changes to the situation such as a break. Burnout is not a diagnosis with validated treatment options. For this reason, if your child is suffering with mood changes that impact their daily life, I strongly recommend they are seen by a clinician who can do a thorough evaluation and provide an appropriate diagnosis and treatment options.

When you've developed a thoughtful plan for your child and they refuse, it can be maddening. As a parent, you are working so hard to get them the help they need, and you know it's important. But as frustrating as it might be, remember that we ask a lot of children facing challenges. Sometimes, rather than talking about their feelings, children will show you how they are feeling by acting out, misbehaving, talking back, or refusing important treatments. While it can seem like they are antagonizing you, remember that it's not a reflection on your parenting, but rather your child struggling to adapt to their plan. In the next chapter, we'll discuss medical trauma—which is common and an underrecognized cause of resistance.

Before we move on, as you reflect on your child's resistance, consider:

- Have you been thinking about your child's resistance as their problem or your problem?
- If you approach the behavior with curiosity, what could you learn about the root cause?
- Which new strategies come to mind?
- Are there ways to give the child more input and control over what they face?
- Does your child seem burnt-out? Can they have a break or more time for fun?
- Is the resistance stemming from an underlying mental health concern like anxiety or depression?

CHAPTER 11

Unpacking Trauma and Protecting Joy

Carlos complained of frequently feeling out of breath. He would become winded on the walk to school and going up the stairs to his third-grade classroom, and he frequently complained of pain and fatigue. He struggled with focus and stamina through the school day. When his family sought me out for treatment, I asked what Carlos's life outside of school was like. It turns out, Carlos was not allowed to run, get sweaty, laugh really hard, or go outside in the spring, summer, or fall. With all these restrictions on his physical activity, it was not surprising he had limited endurance for physical activity.

Carlos had severe asthma as a toddler and was hospitalized in the intensive care unit multiple times. The family knew that seasonal allergies and exercise triggered his asthma, and so these rules were put in place to protect him—they credited these precautions with his survival. But when I was seeing him, nearly five years after his last hospitalization, he had only used an inhaler a handful of times in the past few months. He did not have problems with wheezing or cough. Recently, when he felt out of breath and used the asthma inhaler, he found no difference in his symptoms, likely because his symptoms were related to exertion (i.e., running up the stairs) rather than asthma. The rest of his history, his exam, and testing did not suggest he still had asthma, much less poorly controlled or high-risk asthma.

While parents often see their doctors when their children are in crisis, they rarely have dedicated visits when things are going better to facilitate resuming regular life with confidence. Carlos and his family would have benefited from these types of visits to help steadily and confidently ease up the restrictions they had placed on his lifestyle. It's not that physicians don't see the value in counseling through this process; rather, it's hard to predict which families will want or need the transition assistance. Since these visits aren't preventive, they may not be fully covered by insurance and require time away from school or work, so most doctors may not require them. But this doesn't mean doctors aren't happy to provide the service to families who will find it helpful. Often when things are stable or going well, families feel the support wind down and interpret this to mean that they must figure things out on their own going forward.

For Carlos's family, I could see how scared they were for his well-being and in our conversation, I learned that the family would not trust me enough, especially in a first visit, to follow simple advice such as, "Stop restricting his activities." Because they had been through a traumatic experience, we would have to find a way to incorporate the loosening of his restrictions in a way that left the family feeling safe and supported. Carlos and his family had learned that being winded was a danger sign for an impending emergency, but since he had effectively outgrown his asthma, I had to help them relearn that children frequently play hard and laugh hard in a way that makes them out of breath. Taking the fear out of this daily experience would allow him to live a less restricted life and over time help his endurance and stamina.

Survivors of childhood cancer and congenital heart disease frequently experience similar transition stress. While dealing with intensive issues related to chemotherapy or nutrition, these families can be seen by a health-care provider weekly or even more often. Then when a remission is achieved or a surgery is completed, the families graduate from such close monitoring. These families celebrate this transition—they appreciate the implication that the worst is behind them. But they often find their healing isn't complete and the lack of contact with the health team leads to worsening anxiety.

After an intense time, when one's energy is no longer focused and compartmentalized on the problem at hand, the true processing and healing really begins. When we experience a trauma, there is a numbness that enables us to go through the motions and get through a crisis, even a long one. But when the numbness wears off, "normal" begins to set in; there is an emotional reckoning that has to happen. I've seen this pattern recur with mothers after a traumatic birth experience or NICU stay, parents of young children after a hospitalization, and parents who navigate the uncertainty of a diagnostic workup for a new medical condition or disability. Carlos's family had been through a trauma multiple times when his asthma had been so bad they feared for his life. Before I could address his endurance concerns, I had to help them process what they had been through. In this chapter, we'll address how to identify when you or your child have been through a trauma and ways to find the support you need.

Have You Been through a Trauma?

Many families may be unsure: Is what we've faced really a trauma? Some people describe a difference between "big *T*" Trauma and "little *t*" trauma. The former, most obvious Trauma includes abuse, natural disasters, war, and catastrophic accidents. "Little *t*" trauma can be any event that exceeds our capacity to cope or leads to disruptions in function. Interpersonal conflict, divorce, relocation, and bullying are all examples of "little *t*" trauma that can accumulate and lead to distress.

When children face challenges, you can attempt to classify what they experience into "big *T*" and "little *t*" traumas. We might think of "big *T*" Traumas as intensive care unit stays, surgeries that require intense recovery, or children undergoing long-term treatments such as cancer therapies with frequent blood work and infusions. "Little *t*" traumas might include things like blood draws, vaccinations, emergency room visits, ambulance rides, or educational evaluations. Family members, including parents, grandparents, and siblings, may experience these traumas secondhand as well.

However, the size and scale of the inciting events cannot reliably predict whether a child or a parent will perceive it as a trauma and have difficulties functioning. Even though blood draws and IV placement are not life-threatening procedures, a child may perceive them or the restraint and anticipatory fear as life-threatening. Additionally, a child's sensitivity and vulnerability to the trauma matter too. Children who experience recurrent traumas, underlying mental health concerns, limited supports, or dysfunctional coping skills may be more prone to be negatively impacted by what they experience.

Similarly with parents, the context in which you experience an event has a lot to do with how stressful it is. Imagine a first-time parent navigating a baby's first respiratory illness while sleep deprived, facing work stress, or grieving the loss of a loved one. Their perception of that illness will be markedly different from a parent of three children navigating the same illness while well rested and in a fortified state of mind.

On the other end of the spectrum, some children and parents demonstrate remarkable resilience bouncing back from unimaginable situations. I've seen children be put on a ventilator for a few days in the intensive care unit who appear to seamlessly move on and process what they went through while returning to activities and friendships they enjoy. The only way to know who is struggling is to ask.

It's precisely this variability that makes it difficult for systems to provide the support families need. But because the medical and educational systems don't have this robust support integrated, as a caregiving parent you have to advocate for your needs and the needs of your child.

Parents want to protect their children and help them heal and recover from unpleasant, traumatizing experiences. The first step is to know whether or not your child has experienced an event as a trauma.

Common Trauma Symptoms

Jenson, a four-year-old boy, had been hospitalized for a skin infection. His dad was able to stay with him at the hospital, but his mother stayed home to care for his sibling and dog for the four days—his first time away from her. His treatment required several blood draws and IVs, which he tolerated but certainly found uncomfortable.

When he came home, he was not himself. He could no longer sleep in his room alone, and even when he slept with his parents, he awoke several times a night from nightmares. He had to go back to diapers after being potty trained for over a year. He had meltdowns and tantrums that his parents weren't used to. Some of these fits occurred around things that related to his hospital stay, like in anticipation of a follow-up doctor's visit. But some of his tantrums were triggered by unrelated matters. When he played, he was more dependent on his parents, and he was "clingier" in social situations.

When Jenson's parents came for their follow-up appointment, they wondered if their child had been "broken." Could the infection or one of the antibiotics permanently impact his brain and behavior? As they rounded into the second week of this behavior, they wondered if he would ever be the same. All of Jenson's behavior changes could be classified as consistent with a trauma reaction.

While symptoms of a medical trauma can vary substantially, we generally observe that symptoms fall into the following buckets:

* **Mood changes.** Children can withdraw from social situations, appear down or irritable, or have more variability in their mood (they may have a short fuse).
* **Reexperiencing.** Children can perseverate on details about what they have been through, talking about it excessively, drawing it, incorporating it into their play. To some extent this is expected as a child processes what they have been through. However, when it persists for a longer period or dominates their day, excluding other activities, it can be a sign of trauma.
* **Hyperarousal.** Some children can experience panic attacks, feel "jumpy," or have difficulty winding down to rest at night. Disrupted sleep from hyperarousal can further impair their recovery and coping skills.

- **Avoidance.** Some children will avoid talking about or thinking about anything related to what they have been through. This may manifest as refusal to attend necessary appointments, take medications, or interact with providers.

Trauma in an older child can look different. At fifteen, Adrian was in remission from cancer treatments but was having a lot of behavioral issues at home and school—skipping school, not doing his homework, fighting with friends and his mother. At first, his mother and I weren't sure if he was experiencing normal teen angst or whether his acting out was a sign of trauma or mental health concerns. His behavior wasn't triggered by medical issues, nor did it start right after a time of intense treatment. We asked him a lot of questions to try to understand the connection between what he had been through and his problematic behavior, but it wasn't until he was productively engaged in therapy that he opened up about how he found post-treatment life to be more stressful than before, when he was frequently seeing doctors.

Like Adrian, some older children recovering from a trauma can present subtly and may withdraw from their normal activities. Avoidance can be a sign of trauma and a common way children try to cope—if they cannot talk about or think about what they have been through, they can reduce the unpleasant feelings of stress associated with the experience. Similarly, children may complain of somatic symptoms like headaches or stomachaches because they experience the reaction to stress (elevated heart rate, nausea, fatigue) as physically uncomfortable. For Adrian, this was particularly problematic; he would feel his stress physically, but avoid talking to others about it because of a desire to protect his mom from excess worry. Some children may have the sophistication to complain of invasive worries, difficulty sleeping, and inability to focus or function, but others, like Adrian, may not communicate their distress or understand that help is available.

In my experience, most children who endure hospitalization, a surgery, or a scary experience can be thrown off for a few days and show many of these symptoms. When children can resume their normal routines and activities, catch up on sleep, and be comforted by their loved ones, many are able to begin feeling like themselves again within days or weeks. However, some children will not "bounce back."

The children who do not bounce back will continue to have these sorts of symptoms that impair their quality of life and ability to enjoy their normal activities. It's important to say that when extra support is needed, it's not the fault of the children or of their caregiving parents. A child cannot control how their brains respond to the stress they have been through, and even the most loving caregiver cannot always heal this injury without support. Children and caregivers who carry trauma will need the help of someone appropriately trained in supporting individuals who have been through a trauma.

Evidence-Based Options for Confronting Trauma

Trauma is treatable. If you are reading this and realizing that someone in your family seems to fit this description, you should know there are many evidence-based ways to start getting better in as little as four to six sessions with an appropriately trained psychologist. Finding support isn't always easy, but it can be essential.

You can of course connect with peers, other parents, and people on your care team who have been through similar transitions. They may "get it" and provide support. But approaching trauma that's causing distress in an evidence-based way requires a higher level of treatment that only a therapist or psychiatrist can provide. The National Child Traumatic Stress Network[1] has an incredibly informative website where you can find more details about these treatments and connect with a local provider. In the present, let's review some of the broader features of various evidence-based approaches to treating trauma, as it may help as you seek professional help.

Child-Parent Psychotherapy (CPP)

Children under six are typically offered child-parent psychotherapy. In this work, the child and the parent engage in sessions to support and strengthen the relationship between the child and his or her caregiver to restore the child's functioning. CPP relies on attachment theory and integrates psychodynamic, developmental, and cognitive-behavioral theories. While this is an evidence-based treatment approach, it is highly individualized to the family, and due to the difficulties in working with young children—such as keeping their attention on task—the typical course of therapy is longer than some of the alternatives—as long as a year.

Trauma-Focused Cognitive Behavioral Therapy

Trauma-focused cognitive behavioral therapy (TF-CBT) is recommended for children three and up. In TF-CBT, children learn skills to regulate their affect, behavior, and thought patterns. Often children work with a therapist to form a trauma narrative and process what they have been through in a way to improve coping. A typical course of therapy is twelve to twenty-five sessions with parent participation. This treatment has been shown to work well and for diverse populations.

Eye Movement Desensitization and Reprocessing

In eye movement desensitization and reprocessing (EMDR), a therapist works with a child on reconstructing the trauma narrative while directing the child to move their eyes back and forth. In her book *Small Wonders*, Dr. Joan Lovett describes her experiences as a pediatrician using this technique with a variety of children and hypothesizes that the effectiveness of the therapy comes from the patients reexperiencing their trauma in a safe place. The eye movements, rhythmic tapping, or other movements are designed to be soothing and assist in integrating the trauma narrative to promote coping. Though there is evidence to support this therapy, there is also controversy over how important the eye movements are in promoting its efficacy. Proponents of this technique think that the bilateral and rhythmic movements promote adaptive information processing, facilitating the natural healing that desensitizes and reprocesses traumatic memories.

Play Therapy

In child-centered play therapy (CCPT), children who have been through a trauma are brought to a safe and welcoming environment with thoughtfully selected toys and art materials. They are then encouraged to play. Therapists may reflect the child's feelings and allow the child to find ways to communicate and process what they have been through. Since play is the primary work of the child, CCPT is developmentally appropriate and may be more appealing to your child. This type of therapy is common and may be easier to find but does not have the same level of evidence of effectiveness as some of the others mentioned here—that said, this type of therapy can still provide benefits.

Before signing up for a course of therapy, you can interview the provider and ask questions about the techniques they are using and when you can expect improvement. If you do not see improvement, you can consider finding a second opinion or ask your pediatrician for another option, but don't give up hope.

Interventions to Prevent PTSD

Child and family traumatic stress intervention (CFTSI) is an early intervention program designed for children over seven. Treatment begins with four sessions timed at least thirty to forty-five days after a potentially traumatizing event. In studies that have focused on a high-risk population of families who are psychosocially disadvantaged and exposed to a wide range of types of trauma, CFTSI has been shown to decrease risk of later diagnosis with PTSD by 65 percent. Within the therapy there are two main goals: to increase communication between child and caregiver about the child's feelings from the trauma, and to teach specific behavioral skills to enhance coping. If you have a child who has recently been through a "big *T*" Trauma, finding a supportive resource like this may prevent a child from suffering.

Medications

Sometimes, children who show signs of trauma have underlying mental health concerns such as impaired focus from ADHD, depression, anxiety, or post-traumatic stress disorder. In these situations, sometimes you may be encouraged to seek treatment for these underlying conditions with a psychiatrist who may offer medications. I would encourage you to consider this advice and these medications with an open mind, as starting indicated medications promptly may expedite recovery, especially in conjunction with therapy.

I've shared this background on trauma because it's important for parents to be aware of the possibility that trauma is impacting their family. Often, we fail to recognize children who are struggling due to trauma, but if we identify these children, we can connect them with resources to support their recovery. Even if your child doesn't show signs of trauma, awareness that trauma is treatable will help you support others in your community.

As a parent myself, I understand that parents want more for their children than recovery. We hope that our children will have opportunities to thrive and find happiness. Whether you and your child have met criteria for trauma or not, finding a way to be happy and find joy in your day-to-day life is essential.

Promoting Joy

Annie was an athletic five-year-old girl who found joy in physical activity. From soccer to gymnastics, she wanted to try all of the sports she could, and in between scheduled activities, she was always the one climbing to the top of a play structure or into a water fountain by a pool. So, when she broke her leg, her parents were distraught. Certainly, the leg would heal—it was casted and her pain controlled—but how would their family make it through a month when she couldn't do any of the things she loved to do?

Parenting her through this required the parents not just to treat her pain and promote her recovery, but also help her live as full a life as she could despite her injury. Filling the sudden void of her preferred activity seemed daunting, but her parents brought in puzzles, arts and crafts, Lego kits, extra movies, and video chatting with friends. They also found ways to involve her at the playground with her siblings, playing catch and inventing new games involving her temporary wheelchair. These activities helped distract her from what she was missing or what she was dealing with. It wasn't perfect, and still she was upset at times, but they made it through the month.

Helping children find opportunities for joy means finding ways for them to connect with peers, play, enjoy the activities they used to before their challenge, or find new ones. Parents and siblings also deserve to find joy. For parents this can mean carving out space and time for your own hobbies, whether they are productive or leisurely pursuits. Caregiving parents often feel lonely when facing a challenge, not just because of the isolation that comes with their child's condition but also because the connections from pleasurable pastimes have been interrupted. While fitting in more is always a challenge, finding joy has a way of healing pain. Some doctors have theorized that humor could be prescribed as therapeutic. Laughter has been suggested to relieve pain, promote cognitive functioning, boost immunity, protect from heart attacks, and reduce cortisol levels.[2] Deep belly laughs and time spent on relaxation certainly seem to be essential parts of a healthy life, but psychologist Mihaly Csik-szentmihalyi, author of the book *Flow*, would argue there is a science to what defines an "optimal experience."

Typical "flow" experiences may look superficially like any activity—sports, games, art, and hobbies. But when an individual finds the right fit, something that is just the right level of difficulty for their skills, something they truly love that resonates with them, often they lose track of time and are immersed thoroughly in the activity. Rather than finding the experience fatiguing, the individual finds the time invigorating and energizing. Csikszentmihalyi describes the common characteristics of optimal experience as follows: "Concentration is so intense that there is no attention left over to think about anything irrelevant or to worry about problems. Self-consciousness disappears, and the sense of time becomes distorted."

When preparing for this book, I interviewed dozens of parents, some of whom were years past the toughest part of their challenge. When I asked them how they got through that difficult time, a surprising number of them brought up moments related to finding joy or flow. More than one parent referenced a treat, an actual piece of chocolate or a frivolous TV show, that they rewarded themselves with for having made it through the week. Other parents found moments of flow in creation such as gardening, making music or painting, or in exercise, including sports, walking, and yoga. Not surprisingly, children most frequently find flow in the same sorts of activities—imaginative or cooperative play, creative activities like art and building, or immersive sensory experiences such as swinging or splashing. When you or your child have something that you truly love to do, where you lose track of time and feel refreshed rather than exhausted after, lean in to that experience. Finding a flow state can make you feel better, or fully distract and allow time to work its magic.

Whether you and your family are facing a big, scary challenge or a small one, it's possible that you have found it traumatic. Some people will bounce back from traumatic experiences, but for those who do not, once we identify trauma, we can find ways to recover. Part of recovering from the difficult parts of life is finding time and space to embrace the best parts of life—moments of happiness, laughter, and flow. Sometimes we must adjust to a new normal and find creative ways to adapt, but families facing a challenge deserve joy just as much as anyone—perhaps even more than others. As Brené Brown put it, "Joy, collected over time, fuels resilience—ensuring we'll have reservoirs of emotional strength when hard things do happen."[3] Sometimes we may have to advocate for opportunities to experience the positives of life. In the next section, we'll talk about how to make a comprehensive plan you can maintain over time and review some of the most commonly overlooked areas. But first, consider:

- Has your child been through a traumatic event?
- Have you, your co-parent, or your child's siblings been traumatized by watching what your child has been through?
- Does your life have room for moments of joy and flow? What about the lives of your children, co-parent, and others in your inner circle?
- Are the activities you used to love still part of your life? If not, what are the barriers?

PART IV

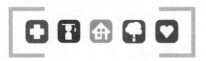

THE LONG RUN

CHAPTER 12

Making a Comprehensive Plan

As I've discussed this book with friends and colleagues over the decade I've been planning it, a lot of people balk at the idea that I can talk generally about challenges. What does addressing depression have in common with food allergies? How can you approach talking about a plan when you don't know what the problem is? But over the years of taking care of children facing a variety of challenges, some trends and themes have emerged.

Regardless of your situation, your plan has to cover a number of bases. The specifics of who, what, and where may change, but good plans tend to be comprehensive:

- A good plan is more than just medication or services.
- A good plan is customized to address the unique needs of the child and the family.
- A good plan understands human nature and creates buffers for human error.

Meanwhile, I've seen many plans fail due to common mistakes:

- A bad plan relies on one person.
- A bad plan relies on strong-arming or bullying.
- A bad plan fails to consider long-term goals and big-picture values.

By now, you hopefully have a sense of what your plan is and what your next steps are. As we approach the end of the book, I'd like to encourage you to take one more look at your plan to consider where the weak spots might be. If we can identify the weak spots early on, we can form a more effective plan, one that you can feel more confident about.

You Really Can't Do It All

Jason and Julia's child seems depressed. Ever since they moved and she's been going through puberty, she is more withdrawn, sleeping more, and expressing less joy. They want to help her right away, and their preference is that they'll form a plan to handle this on their own. While this might sound surprising, it's unfortunately quite common that parents try to handle behavioral health needs on their own—perhaps because of stigma, barriers to care, or a mistaken sense of mental health needs as reflective of inadequate parenting.

Jason is quite knowledgeable about best practices to encourage wellness, promoting good sleep, meditation, and exercise. Julia wants to focus on their child's friendships and hopes to entice her into some of the activities that used to bring her joy. The parents think if they focus on the basics that have worked in the past, hopefully she'll be back on track soon.

Do you see the flaws in this plan? By attempting to handle their daughter's challenges on their own, these parents may have missed something. Without a mental health assessment by a pediatrician, psychiatrist, or therapist, the parents can't know the extent of the depression. What if the child's depression is more severe than they realize and she is considering suicide? What if there has been abuse or drug use that she is scared to discuss with her parents? What if the depressive symptoms continue to worsen?

While a family is an independent unit, and likely used to solving problems and helping its members on its own, when it comes to making a plan, often you need help. Even if Jason and Julia were health professionals in related fields, they would not be the best qualified individuals to help their daughter. Getting a third party involved will provide access to another level of screening, some perspective, and a safe space to promote their child's well-being.

Often, as parents we hesitate to ask for help, but what advice would you give to a friend facing this same challenge? If you were going to recruit more help, consider: What additional resources would you access in an ideal world? Even if you don't want to bring them in now, thinking through what your options will be and what would make you take that next step is important.

Safety Issues

Deirdre's son James has an allergy to nuts. Working with his elementary school had been frustrating—they called her frequently about paperwork and required her to attend every field trip to supervise his safety. Now, as he enters middle school right across the street from their home, he can reliably identify food with nuts. He carries his epinephrine injector, and he hasn't needed to use it in years. "So", Deirdre says, "let's just keep this between us, James, and that way you don't have to bother with the paperwork or the school nurse."

This plan could be tempting; getting the forms completed takes a lot of time and often an extra epinephrine injector for school is expensive and not covered fully by health insurance. For a tween, the burden of looping in the school may seem too great, as they dislike being identified as different, having to check in with the school nurse, or tolerating Mom's supervision on a field trip. However, I can't recommend cutting out the school nurse. Even the most diligent child or adult can have an accidental exposure to an allergen. Are we really going to rely on a twelve-year-old to own the responsibility for having his medication available at all times and having the judgment on when to use it, when the issue hasn't come up in years?

Children venture out from their family bubble often—school-age children spend 28 percent of their daytime hours at school, and accordingly 10–25 percent of injuries occur at school.[1] You can't control the environment absolutely, even if you try. Others are involved even if it would be simpler to do on your own. Take a moment to consider how this scenario might play out. If James should innocently eat candy containing nuts, but Deirdre, although she's across the street, is busy with work and misses the call from school—which doesn't have his epinephrine—they will call 911. The ambulance comes and gives epinephrine, but the delay causes James's initial symptoms to progress and he now has to be admitted to the hospital for management.

Although the odds of something like this happening are small, it's worthwhile to spend the energy and money to put a good emergency plan in place. It may not seem warranted, based on how unlikely it is that your child has a reaction on the day they have forgotten their epinephrine *and* you aren't around. But it could happen.

It's uncomfortable to consider worst-case scenarios, especially concerning your child. Even the most conscientious parents sometimes avoid spending time on this because they somehow fear this will make the worst-case scenario more likely to happen. But making a plan to address these issues can improve your confidence and potentially help you relax. As you consider what to include in your plan, you do not have to start from scratch.

The Emergency Information Form (EIF) was developed by the American Academy of Pediatrics and the American College of Emergency Physicians.[2] In addition to the care plan details we drafted earlier, with contact information for the doctors and a medication list, the EIF adds a section for contingencies and drills. Contingencies include your child's common problems—perhaps your child has had recurrent urinary tract infections—on the form, you'd jot down the typical symptoms and what has worked best in the past. While "drills" may seem extreme, considering what you would do in case of some possible scenarios such as power loss, a flood, or a water safety issue may prompt you to take action to prepare in advance.

Supervision

Jessica's four-year-old son has dysphagia—difficulty swallowing things correctly. Jessica and her partner first learned he was unable to swallow safely after he experienced several severe back-to-back pneumonias when he was a baby. Because of his anatomy, when he was an infant, he would drink milk and some would spill into his lungs, causing both irritation (chemical pneumonitis) and bacterial infection (pneumonia). Once we identified the cause and found another way to hydrate him—by a feeding tube—he stopped having pneumonias. While he is making slow and steady progress in feeding therapy, he has not been able to drink thin liquids safely. He can eat many foods and textures by mouth, but still gets water through his feeding tube. While Jessica takes him weekly to feeding therapy, this school year he began taking the bus and his babysitter watches him after school, since Jessica works late.

When Jessica's son first came down with another pneumonia, we attributed it to a virus and figured he'd caught it through the exposure to other kids at preschool. But when the second pneumonia came up, we thought it may be related to his swallowing and we started talking about repeating his swallowing study to be sure his swallowing skills hadn't worsened. We were talking about this in the exam room while he played, but he was listening in. "Oh, Mommy," he said, "my swallowing has gotten better. I'm even able to drink a juice box now!" The mom's eyebrows rose and her cheeks turned red. We subsequently learned that on the bus his seatmate had been sharing his apple juice on the way home. The bus driver and attendant didn't know this was off-limits, though children generally weren't supposed to eat or drink on the bus.

Once they knew to stop the juice boxes, his breathing issues improved, but I share the anecdote to remind you to continue to supervise the important stuff. When you are managing a team, it's essential to keep checking in with the babysitter, bus driver, and teachers regularly about important issues.

Even supervising your family remains important. If your child is managing their own daily medication, you should continue to ensure it's taken regularly by keeping track of refills or observing them taking their medications every once in a while. While we do want to foster independence, we want to acknowledge that the developing child may underestimate the importance of taking their medication and need help.

Take a moment to consider your strategy for supervising the stakeholders involved in your children's life. We want to ensure that if your bus driver has a concern about something, they have a way to communicate with you, and vice versa. As you supervise your child, you also have an opportunity to be a coach. So, building in questions when you check in like "How's this going for you?" will open doors for you to learn about things you might not have otherwise.

Opening the dialogue to your family and caregiving team will be important as well to keep your plan in tip-top shape and also foster connection.

Promoting Social and Emotional Well-Being

My teenage patient had a flat affect—she wasn't smiling, and her voice was monotone. Despite her pink hair and spunky sense of style, Eileen didn't talk about her friends or passions like most teenagers who visited my office. Even before we got to the part of the well-child visit where I spoke to her alone, my instincts told me that she was depressed. Being a teenager is hard on anyone, and her teen years were also colored by a craniofacial abnormality and a tracheostomy tube. The tube involved a small white tube that went from her neck into her airway to help her breathe. Medically she was doing quite well, gaining independence in her care and staying healthy and up-to-date, but I was worried about her well-being.

She had been my patient for a few years; typically, we chatted about her support system, activities, school, and friends just like every other child would. Sometimes we would chat about the ways in which her care needs impacted her life—the inconvenience of needing a nurse on the first overnight school trip, the disruption of not being able to swim at camp (water might enter her airway due to the tracheostomy tube), and the isolation of being excluded by the popular kids at school due to her differences. Precisely because she would open up to me, her parents, and her school counselor about such stresses, and because she also mentioned finding her place, a few close friends, and some passions, I had hoped she would be okay. Retrospectively, I wondered if I could have asked different questions or helped in some way to avoid reaching this point, and I'm sure her mom did too. But we can't always predict or prevent when the biochemistry, hormones, genetic risks, and environmental stressors will align to lead to depression. Now that we identified her depression, we could start treatment—for her, this consisted of both an antidepressant and seeing a psychiatrist in addition to the prior supportive therapy she had received at school. Her symptoms improved.

While this collision of factors and depression can be a part of any teen's life, the added mental and emotional strain of facing a challenge increases one's risk. When a child has a mental health challenge such as depression, there is no substitute for professional help in forming a treatment plan. However, all parents want to promote their child's emotional health. If your child is doing well, you want to keep them well. Parents facing a challenge should ask: What can we do proactively to promote resilience and coping?

In the next section, I'll share some strategies parents can use to load the toolbox of resilience, but it's essential to understand that mental health struggles are not always preventable. Even if you do everything "right" as a parent, your child may need additional support. Some parents may feel very deep pain when their child is struggling, so it's especially important for them to know that while our behaviors affect our well-being, biochemistry and genetics sometimes have a larger impact.

Connection

Families facing a challenge commonly face isolation and stigma, whether their challenge involves a disability or a disease. In *Raising a Rare Girl*,

Heather Lanier discusses raising her disabled daughter Fiona. "Normal is not just a range on the bell curve. It's also a community, a collective. To be Normal is to partake in a certain kind of belonging with others. This was one thing that made parenting Fiona unexpectedly hard—the isolation of difference. We could not relate to other parents and their children. They could not often relate to us."

One of the most important things we can do to promote our children's well-being is to help them feel connected to others. We know that having safe, stable, nurturing relationships is one of the biggest predictors of resilience. However, it can be more difficult for children who have a challenge or who are different to form close relationships and connections.

What strategies can we use to promote connections in our children? First, we can be more conscious of how our choices impact our children's friendships. Parents can help by simply identifying friendships as a family priority. We have to acknowledge that the relationships may come from unexpected places. Some children make friends at school, but others find connection in other community institutions like art class, the library, or church. Some children, particularly when facing something big, connect with peers facing similar challenges through summer camps or programs for their condition.

Wherever these friendships come from, recognize them as valuable assets to your children's well-being and facilitate them as you are able. For some, this may mean going out of your way to help the kids see each other despite the inconvenience or facilitating a video chat or playdate to stay in touch.

If your child is having trouble finding friends, I'd encourage you to keep trying. Katrina Ubell, a pediatrician who has established a coaching business to help busy health-care providers, describes the goal of finding friends as similar to filling a job opening. To find the right match, you might have to interview a lot of different applicants. Sometimes you'll get lucky and find the right one right away, but other times it may take dozens or even hundreds of attempts before you click with the right person.

That said, if your child is struggling to form close relationships with others despite many exposures to potential friends, it's worth checking in with your educational or medical support team for ideas. Some children may take more support to develop positive relationships, such as repeated exposures and modeling to learn how to form positive relationships. Some psychologists and occupational therapists run facilitated playgroups because kids can be helped along in their executive function and communication skills. With those skills, children can develop rich and fulfilling relationships.

A Positive Sense of Self

Martin Seligman has established the field of positive psychology, oriented toward not just preventing crisis but also helping promote happiness. In his book *Flourish*, he lays out the basics of what someone needs to be happy: to experience pleasure, to engage in a flow state, and to feel your life has meaning.

While this may feel abstract, I find that parents do the first two with their children by default. We notice what our children enjoy and help them to find more positive experiences. We expose our children to activities, environments, and toys designed to help promote their engagement. But the last one—helping your child to find meaning—is something we rarely discuss.

When I asked families to explain how they coped with a long-term challenge, they did find meaning in their own ways. In the process of grasping how the challenge impacted their child's identity and their own, they were able to understand themselves better and find meaning in their stories.

One parent said: "Having a child with a disability has been hard, harder than I ever could have imagined honestly. But I've also learned through this experience that I am stronger and more capable than I would have thought. Now, when I can help moms new to this condition to get there a little faster, it seems to all make sense."

Another told me: "What our family went through with our son's condition and the associated long hospital stays was so challenging—for him, for me, and for my other children. And what eventually helped us to heal was to find meaning in the experience. For us, we've been able to engage in advocacy and give back to the community of people who've been impacted by this diagnosis."

While these families have the luxury of being past the acute crisis of their experience, what they share is that they have integrated their experience into their story. Our challenges shape us in ways that we expect and ways we don't. My own experience having cancer made me who I am today, a doctor who has a lot of empathy for the lived experience of families outside of the clinic and hospital setting. My story led me to become someone who finds meaning in helping others.

We can't fast-forward through the hard stuff to this kind of acceptance, but we can help form our children's positive sense of self and identity. Often when facing a challenge, our children show us their unique skills and characteristics. By highlighting their strengths, we can help them to build their positive identity.

Frequently I've seen challenges bring out these strengths:

- Humor
- Patience
- Kindness
- Empathy
- Determination
- Creativity
- Optimism

These strengths, and others you may identify, are like little seeds, and recognizing them is like watering them and exposing them to sunlight. It will help them to blossom and become a part of the narrative. If possible, try to see the strengths your child and others in your family bring to the challenge.

Writing Our Own Story

For many families, isolation occurs out of necessity. The logistic or practical challenges associated with your challenge seem insurmountable and there is not enough time, money, or energy for finding space to connect with people outside the household. Other families hesitate to put themselves out there for fear of rejection, judgment, or pity.

The truth is that as parents, we can only control so much in our child's environment. We can try to educate those in our community, but when leaving the bubble of the home environment, there is always an unpredictable element. We can't say how knowledgeable the strangers, acquaintances, and individuals in your community are about your child's condition. People will say the wrong thing even if they are well-intentioned. There's no way to avoid these situations entirely.

We talked in Chapter 9 about how you can roll with these situations as a parent, but how can you help your child cope with unwelcome or unkind messages from others? The first strategy is perhaps the most basic: we can write our own story.

Imagine that you're at the playground with your son who has cerebral palsy and uses braces and sometimes assistive devices to get around. At the park, a girl invades his personal space and asks a lot of questions about "what's wrong" with him. Later, at dinner, your co-parent asks about your outing and your child is busy eating. You have an opportunity to narrate the experience.

One option is to ignore or minimize the negative experience. This sets the example that yes, while it happened, it wasn't the focus of how you spent your afternoon. You can choose to focus on other parts of your day and let it go. If you feel like your son was bothered by the experience, always making this type of choice probably wouldn't be the best choice, because he may want to talk about it.

If you decide you do want to describe the experience, there is a broad range of things you could say.

You might say, "This mean girl got right up in our space and wouldn't leave us alone. She was going on and on about the braces and walker. It totally ruined our time at the park." This may reflect the truth of how you experienced the interaction and may help validate your son's uncomfortable feelings, but it also risks encouraging your son to view uneducated people in your community as a threat and as violators looking to make him feel bad.

Or you could say, "We had fun, but we met a girl who had never even met a child who used braces before. How strange to get to be eight years old and have never met anyone like our son." This technique encourages your family to understand other people's perspective and see unwelcome or unkind behavior as *their* problem, not your problem.

Or you could say, "It was a nice day at the park, but there was another child who was asking a lot of questions." Then you might ask your son, "How was that for you?" This opens the door for your son to share how it made him feel. If your child is able to open up, you may be surprised to learn how their experience of a situation differs from yours.

Some children have transition points where they are likely to experience more of this friction—a child returning to school after a long absence, a child entering a mainstream classroom after years of special education, or a child with a visible disability in a new environment. If your child is in a school setting, you may have access to resources such as a school counselor or dedicated teacher who can check in with your child. Taking advantage of these third-party individuals can be very helpful.

I've heard from many children that they want to protect their parents from the hard things they encounter. Sometimes they may fear that if things aren't going well and they complain to you, school may be taken away or changed for the worse. Sometimes children assume you won't get it, and you may not fully understand the context. If you know the classroom dynamic or the personalities involved, you can often see peer behavior in a different light.

If your child goes through an experience that is really troubling, upsetting, or even traumatizing, I recommend that you seek help in making a plan to help them through it. Showing your child love, making them feel safe, and helping them resume their normal routines are some things that will encourage coping. While it is tempting to want to talk to your child a lot about their experience in the days to weeks following, it's likely better to follow your child's cues. Forcing a child to talk about an uncomfortable memory can consolidate the memory and worsen flashbacks. Child-life therapists, social workers, psychologists, and psychiatrists have additional training on helping children process acute traumas.

Anticipating What's to Come

Samantha's son Henry has recently been diagnosed with a learning disability. He has a solid Individualized Education Plan (IEP) at school with multiple types of supports, and the pediatrician got involved to do a developmental assessment, check his hearing and vision, and ensure there weren't other complicating issues. It seems like there is a good plan in place, but Samantha still feels unsettled. When I ask her why, it's because she's uncertain about the future. What happens if the IEP doesn't work to help him stay on grade level? What if he has social and emotional difficulties coping with the diagnosis? What will she do if he experiences bullying because of his learning differences? While they have a solid plan in place, she doesn't have confidence that she has identified all the resources he might need if things get worse.

Some of this is natural anxiety that all parents feel regarding the unpredictable nature of raising a child. You can't possibly anticipate all the future needs, and some of the mantras we spoke of earlier can be helpful when these types of worries intrude. Coping with anxiety is part of being an effective caregiver.

However, you can also review your plan to consider some future scenarios. The practical side of worrying is that it allows you to prepare for multiple contingencies.

Samantha could ask her school team when she should expect improvements, and what the plan would be if this doesn't help. She could ask other parents in the community what schools have best addressed their children's special learning needs. This research builds your practical fund of knowledge and can help you feel more prepared for whatever comes. Another way to look at your plan is to ask:

- Am I planning for success? How will I know it and what will change at that point?
- Am I planning for "failure"? If this intervention doesn't go well, what will the next step be?
- If I was telling a friend what to do, would I recommend they consider resources that I'm not taking advantage of?

Taking the time to imagine the broad range of what could be will help you plan most effectively. Maybe you should apply to a different school for next year if your child's trajectory seems to be on track for thriving in an environment with more or less support. Maybe you need to financially plan now to prepare in case your child's condition worsens and requires a leave of absence from your job.

When we first make plans, the priority is to address current identified needs. But thinking broadly about what may be coming can enable us to make a more comprehensive plan. In a year or two when you look back at where you are today, what will you wish you spent more time on or less time on? Change is the only constant in parenting, and caregiving is no different. Changing needs, changing environments, and changing preferences all require us to be flexible and think on our feet

To make a comprehensive, high-quality plan is an overwhelming task. So, while I'll try to help you think of everything, I'd also like to reassure you that a good-enough plan is an adequate goal.

––––––––

In this chapter, we've reviewed the importance of ensuring you have enough support, prioritizing safety, continuing supervision, thinking about the future, and considering your child's social and emotional well-being as you make your plan. We can help our children form robust connections with others, cultivate a positive sense of a self, and allow them to narrate their own story. These techniques are useful for all children, but when children face a challenge, these proactive measures matter even more.

In the next chapter, we'll talk about ways to build and maintain motivation over time. Before you move on, consider:

- Does your plan depend too much on one person to be sustainable?
- Are there areas where your child needs ongoing supervision or support?
- What are you doing to promote your child's social and emotional adjustment?
- In the long term, what's the most important part of the plan?
- If things worsen, what will you need?
- If things improve, what will be the next steps?

CHAPTER 13

Maintaining Motivation

While looking at photos, William's mom noticed that her son's head was tilted a little bit to the right in every photo. When she brought this to my attention, I recommended he see an eye doctor, who confirmed Mom's inkling that something was off—William had strabismus, or an abnormal alignment of the eyes. Moreover, the strabismus was likely due to the fact that his vision in one eye was much stronger than the vision in the other eye. Mom left the visit with a box of patches and a plan to cover up his good eye for at least two hours a day.

Since William was four, mom suspected that this task would not be easy. But after she read some tips on a Facebook group, she found and ordered patches with his favorite cartoon characters, and the first few days went surprisingly fine. Whether it was the character or the novelty of the whole situation, William went along with it at first.

But after a week, the eye patches lost their appeal. The adhesive made him itch and he felt like he couldn't play as well when he couldn't see from both eyes. He had started to notice the extra attention the patch drew from other kids at the playground or grocery store—not the kind of attention he wanted.

At this point, his mom called me and asked what she could do to help him stay motivated to complete the course of therapy. She knew if he didn't follow the instructions, he risked permanent vision loss and the alternatives to the patch weren't a good fit according to his doctor. But he was not a toddler anymore and she sensed that strong-arming him into wearing the patch might backfire and worsen his resistance.

Chronic challenges will inherently have ups and downs. If our children have a long-lasting challenge, or when parents are balancing multiple priorities, it goes without saying that at times our focus will be elsewhere. This may be because the other parts of your life need attention or are intentionally the priority.

Or it may be that you or your child are deeply tired of dealing with a challenge. Many challenges require a lot of work, requiring physical diligence and mental energy that can be exhausting. Parents often feel guilty or anxious about this waning motivation, but if we can acknowledge this difficulty as part of the process and as something to be expected, we can make a better plan for facing it.

Lack of motivation doesn't mean that you or your child are lazy. Many people who don't face challenges struggle to motivate themselves to do the work of taking care of their body—to drink and eat healthful amounts, to move their body frequently, or to sleep enough. When you face a challenge, the demands on your time and energy are above and beyond these typical needs. Developing strategies to stay engaged in the necessary work will help you face your challenge. In the remainder of the chapter, we'll discuss strategies to maintain motivation for you and your child.

Maximize Intrinsic Motivators

Intrinsic motivators are things you do because they are fun, enjoyable, or satisfying. When these tasks are done, they satisfy a basic psychological need—to feel independent, competent, or loved. For a child like William, patching was probably engaging at first because he could pick the patch, place it on his eye, and do so with his mom, whom he loves. Over time this motivation waned, but by thinking about what got him to do it in the first place, you can think about strategies to get him to continue to do it.

When a child is able to view a task, even an undesirable one, as meaningful and important to their higher goals, they will be much more motivated to complete it.[1] Some children will be able to say, "Taking care of myself matters and so I will be vigilant about working toward this goal." Many children, especially four-year-olds, won't be able to engage in that sort of long-term planning, but we can coach children to see other intrinsic reasons to participate. Imagine William's mom saying, "I know you are really good at listening and paying attention, so later when your father asks you to put on your patch, I bet you will listen!" In a way this ties the desired behavior to something the child already sees as part of their identity. Another motivator can be pleasure—a task that is associated with positive things like connection, music, dance, or play will be easier for a child to embrace. Here are some examples of things you could try.

- His older brother, someone he admires and seeks attention from, could place the patch every day and follow this with a hug. Putting the patch on may become something he does with his brother, making the task inherently more special.
- After he puts a patch on himself, he could put a patch on one of his stuffed animals. Or, if you have old photos or books, you could give him stickers or allow him to "patch" some of the people he sees. This would foster feelings of agency and independence.
- To utilize his competitive instinct, you could make a habit of hiding the patch in the kitchen every morning, and whichever family member finds it first wins.
- Some children might connect with the idea that they are exercising their eye, and if they keep up the hard work the eye will get stronger. Perhaps you can encourage a sense of gratitude by noting small progress toward reaching a goal.

For some children, maximizing these intrinsic motivating factors may not seem to work. With many strategies to maintain motivation, some may seem to work for a while and then fade, but the benefit of incorporating intrinsic motivators is that they encourage the child to develop a positive sense of self. William is a boy who can do hard things when he needs to. William is a boy who can take responsibility for something important. Even once the patches are no longer necessary, William may internalize these positive messages.

For parents, remembering the purpose and underlying goal of the task can help us maintain focus. We can try to remind ourselves of this with statistics or facts—the doctor said that if we do this for six months, he may not need surgery. Some parents are reminded of the meaning behind their work when they mentor others—one of the unexpected benefits of spending time with individuals newly diagnosed with your child's condition is that it reminds you of all that you've learned and accomplished and can fuel your continued efforts.

Consider External Motivators

If you were to say to William, "Every time you put on an eye patch, you get a piece of chocolate," this would be an example of an extrinsic motivator. You do the activity for an external gain—a reward, acknowledgment, power, or to avoid a consequence. External motivators have been out of vogue in the last few years. Many experts now advise against them, because praise and rewards will, over time, reduce your child's willingness to work hard on their own.

However, as Melinda Moyer explains in her book, *How to Raise Kids Who Aren't Assholes*, much of the research this is based on is somewhat specific. One study, for example, paid college students to do puzzles that were relatively fun to do. When they stopped paying them, the students did less of them than the group who was never paid to do the puzzles. While this tells you that rewards can decrease motivation, it doesn't necessarily apply to things that aren't fun. There are many times when external motivators can be useful tools at helping a child do something unpleasant.

The classic example is a sticker chart. If you do your patching, you'll get a sticker. Earn ten or thirty stickers and you can have a movie night or a trip to the toy store. For many children, an external motivator like this can be exciting.

As adults, we think of ourselves as being past sticker charts, but the truth is that there can be benefits to using rewards to motivate us to work through undesirable work. Maybe you are really dreading helping your child through a colonoscopy prep, for example. You can link the unpleasant task with a reward, like ordering delivery from your favorite restaurant. The anticipation of the prize can help you get geared up for the task at hand. I've spoken to many parents who viewed a special piece of chocolate, a walk with a friend, or a favorite TV show as positive anchors of their week.

Over time, rewards become less interesting and can be overdone. You may find that over time the child requires more and more to feel motivated, and you may need to pivot to offer another incentive. So, I would recommend using rewards selectively.

Rewards are not the only external motivators. Avoiding judgment or punishment is another type of external motivator. A child who doesn't want to take their medicine may do so when they know that Dad will be upset if they do not. A child who doesn't want to do their homework may choose to do so when they consider that their teacher will be upset if they do not. This type of motivation long-term can erode trust and interfere with the kinds of connections we want to foster with our children.

Sometimes people lack motivation simply because they are overwhelmed by a demand—an upcoming surgery, a big project that will require a lot of effort, or the sheer number of chronic demands that can't be delayed or skipped. If your motivation is low because you are dealing with so much, consider some ways to make matters less overwhelming.

Take a Thoughtful Break

Rest is restorative. If you are truly just so tired of fighting with your child about wearing an eye patch or taking their medication every day, consider taking a break. Sometimes your doctor may be able to safely say, "Take a few days off." If that's not a reasonable option, see if you can find someone else to handle it. Not necessarily forever—but if your co-parent, grandparent, babysitter, school nurse, or anyone else can take it on just for a few days, the chore may feel more manageable when you return to it. A break can also give you a chance to interrupt a power struggle or a negative cycle of behavior. You can gain a new perspective on why it was bothering you so much and find a new way to approach the task.

Break Down Big Goals

Sometimes big projects can be so overwhelming, we want to put them off or procrastinate. For example, perhaps your child has special educational needs and physical disabilities. The process of finding the right school may feel overwhelming. You have a lot of options, numerous factors to consider, extensive research to do, and it's going to be important to your family's long-term happiness. Going on tours, discussing the schools with the preschool team and other families, and doing the applications and evaluations necessary can easily consume over a hundred hours of work.

If you break this complex project down into steps, you can check off a list; then you can instead focus on one discrete task at a time to make it more manageable:

- Step 1: Create a list of schools and ask your community for others to consider.
- Step 2: Develop a list of what you need in your ideal school.
- Step 3: Create a list of questions to ask about how each school can accommodate your child.
- Step 4: Tour and research the schools on your list.
- Step 5: Bring your favorites back to your family and core care team to seek their input.

Hopefully, each task feels more manageable because there are concrete steps that can be accomplished in a reasonably fixed time and checked off the list. Some parents might feel better breaking it down even further and scheduling blocks of time on their calendar such as, "During each of my child's naps this week, I will call and get information on one school." A project like applying to school can be amorphous, but when you simplify the steps and pace it out, you can stay on target to complete the process on the necessary timeline. If you fall behind schedule, you can also ask for help in accomplishing the next necessary step.

Lean on Your Community, Lean on Your Team

As I spoke with families who had faced challenges, one thing I heard again and again was the benefit of mentorship. While we expect that the one receiving the advice also receives the benefit, what I heard from families was often about the benefit of giving advice. When you give advice to others who may be facing similar things, it provides an opportunity for you to reflect on what you have accomplished and see the bigger picture of your challenge. These discussions highlight the underlying reasons for your goals and actions, and the process of finding meaning in this way can lead to feeling more motivation.

Your peers and your child's peers are not the only individuals who can support these types of discussions. Often, at the beginning of a challenge, families reach out to therapists, teachers, and medical-team members for guidance and clarification. But over time, parents gain confidence and stop reaching out. Inevitably things come up, and their instinct becomes to handle them on their own.

One of the families in my care had three children with sickle cell, ranging from eight to thirteen years old. Frequently, when children with sickle cell get sick, dehydrated, or cold, their blood cells can change shape, leading to painful episodes. The children's disease was on the mild end of the spectrum of severity, and the family had avoided the hospital since the kids were young because the parents knew how to handle minor pain events and keep them from progressing with over-the-counter pain medication, hydration, proper clothing, and other interventions.

But as the eldest became more athletic and independent and started puberty, she began having more sickle cell issues. The pain that had previously struck maybe three times a year started to occur every month and then nearly every week. When they finally came in to discuss this, I gave them a little bit of a hard time. I had wanted to know about her worsening symptoms sooner so that I could help. Just because they had gotten into the habit of handling things on their own didn't mean that I couldn't continue to support their family.

As the parent, you know your child best and you should be proud of your competence in supporting your child. But don't forget there are others ready to help. Sometimes they may not contribute much, but often they will bring a different perspective to enrich and improve your child's care.

———

Maintaining motivation is one of the most important advanced parenting skills. There will be a time, hopefully when you may not be as engaged with medical and educational professionals. During this phase, when you're just living life with your child's challenge, it will be necessary to keep motivation up long-term.

Many times, a family can find ways to use a child's strengths to keep them going. Imagine a child with learning disabilities struggling in school. Perhaps you can use their sense of humor to relieve frustration. You can compliment them on their stamina or perseverance when they work hard. If they are competitive, you can encourage practicing skills by making it into a game they can win or attempt to complete faster. When you work with your child's personality, you'll likely have more success than when you implement your own ideas, and noticing their strengths will help them develop drive and positive self-regard. Sometimes, using external motivators like rewards and praise can be helpful tools too. Big picture, understanding when we need to take a break and when to ask for support are other essential skills that help us to advocate for our families and build out a plan that fits with our values and priorities.

As we move past this section, consider:

- What has worked best to motivate you and your family in the past?
- Are there intrinsic motivators that you might have underestimated?
- Have you tried rewards, praise, and other extrinsic motivators? When did this work well and when did it not?
- If you are feeling overwhelmed, can you take a break? Can a big goal be deconstructed into smaller, more manageable objectives?
- Do you think someone on your care team could help?

CONCLUSION

When I was still a doctor in training, I met an eight-year-old boy named Bryan. Recently, he had started wetting the bed after years without incident. His parents thought maybe it was a behavior issue, but within a few days noticed that he was drinking a huge amount of water. They tried to limit his intake, but he was very thirsty. He seemed pale, flushed, and tired, like he might have been getting sick, and then he started vomiting. They thought maybe he had a stomach bug, but he didn't have a fever and no one else was sick. When he complained of abdominal pain, they were concerned it might be appendicitis and brought him to the emergency room.

There he was promptly diagnosed with a severe presentation of type 1 diabetes. He was admitted to the hospital for a few days for intravenous fluids and insulin to stabilize his electrolytes and blood sugar. In a whirlwind fifty hours, he and his parents received intensive teaching on how to manage his diabetes at home. It was my job to review his discharge plan. We went over the upcoming appointments and the medication plan, which included checking his blood sugar every three hours and the precautions for identifying dangerously low blood sugars. I reviewed how to call and ask for help if needed. I asked, "Do you have any questions?" The dad, his eyes wide and his hands shaky, said, "Just one. How will we sleep again?" While they wanted to go home, leaving the hospital meant taking on a huge new responsibility.

For this family and for many, there is a gap. On one side is the medical or educational plan and on the other end there is the family's life. Throughout this book, my purpose has been to support you as a caregiving parent in bridging that gap. I hope the resources offered can function like a road map to help you navigate your challenge with confidence and find the answers and support you need.

We started by understanding what you bring to the challenge—your strengths, your priorities, and the details of the system in which you're operating. Then we talked about how to effectively research your child's condition, how to learn new skills to support your caregiving, and to take inventory of the rest of your family. We tackled all the hard feelings parents confront when facing a challenge, how to work with your child, and how to promote their well-being. We ended with reviewing the most common things forgotten in otherwise good plans and ways to maintain motivation.

If you are feeling overwhelmed and wondering what comes next, remember you do not have to figure it out all at once or attempt to get it all "right." Part of what's disorienting about helping your child in a challenge is that each family and each child is so unique; rather than finding *the* best way forward, you want to find *your* best way forward. You may find that this book works best as a living resource—topics that didn't seem so important or quite make sense today may seem more relevant in six months or a year.

The work you are doing to support your family and to advocate for your children is important and has value. By seeing the enormous impact parents can have on their children's well-being, I hope you are reminded of the importance of your contribution. The confidence that comes from knowing your worth and feeling prepared to meet your child's challenge can help you speak up.

Often the school, therapists, doctors, and hospitals see things from a different perspective, but most of the individuals in those institutions want to align with your goals and help your children. If the system is not working for you, it's quite likely that it's not working for others. It's the "squeaky wheels" who catch the attention of those involved, and only then will things begin to change.

As a parent, particularly one who is so thoughtful as to dedicate the time and energy to read this book, you are the expert on your child, and you are the customer. Yes, doctors and other experts you may consult have knowledge, experience, and resources you do not, but you bring so much to the table. Think of yourself as a peer to these professionals and express your needs clearly despite the barriers and biases of our systems. Developing your voice to work as partners will be a huge benefit to your child.

Underlying this is advocacy. You may think of advocacy as an endeavor you have no time, energy, or space for. You may think, "I am only trying to help my child." But in your path to help your child and your family, it's inevitable that things will come up where your work can help others, either as an example or by promoting change.

One of my most sophisticated parents invested weeks researching the local laws and Medicaid policies with the goal of having a wheelchair lift installed in her home. She did not think about other children in this process. She thought about meeting her family's immediate needs. When she proudly showed us the photos of the final product, the doctors and social workers took notes. In the end, what we learned from her process we were able to share with others to more effectively help them. Her work helped at least another dozen families get the equipment they needed in the following year alone. So, even if you aren't intending to be an advocate, it's possible you already are one.

Currently our society views parenting as a universal shared experience but doesn't include the many parents who act as a caregiver in addition to being a parent. Considering that nearly a third of children in the United States are living with a chronic medical condition (and this percentage is increasing), caregiving for children is part of the universal experience of being a parent.

I hope that now you see there is a big community of parents like you, who are supporting their children in these essential ways. I have learned not to compliment parents who go above and beyond to support their children in difficult times. While I am so inspired by the dedication, tirelessness, selflessness, and thoughtfulness many parents show day to day, I have learned that many perceive these compliments as a veiled insult.

Many times, a parent will interrupt a compliment to say, "I'm just doing what any parent would do." To imply that their parenting journey is so different than that of any other parent is to put up barriers that do more harm than good. We are all parents doing the best we can for our children. Sometimes, we may take things to another level and use another skill set—advanced parenting—but it's all part of the same experience.

Parents—even ones who have children who are not facing challenges—are better off hearing these stories and learning some of these skills required. We like to be prepared for any issue that may arise, but more importantly, understanding what families face allows you to be a supportive neighbor, a good boss, a helpful aunt or uncle, and a thoughtful member of your community. This literacy for what families face also allows us to teach our children how to be kind, inclusive individuals who make things better.

Once we see the world through this lens, we can talk about the fact that the wheelchair accessible pathway at the zoo involves an extra mile of walking, or notice that at the airport there is no clean and reasonable place to change a child's diaper if they are too heavy for a changing table. If you look around your place of worship, your mall, or your community center, and you don't see individuals with special health-care needs, you can stop and question if there are barriers to their inclusion. This evolution will make us better.

If you take nothing else away from this book, I hope you remember that you aren't alone. Parents are all united in their love and dedication to their children. Whether you are parenting a typical child through typical problems or a unique child through a rare, complex diagnosis, you are using the same toolbox of skills. The process of research, communication, coping, and advocating for your family entails the same sort of work, the same skills, and the same endurance. We are all doing the best we can to support the people we love.

The essential aspects of who we are can be fundamentally formed by our challenges, but when we reframe challenges as being part of life, expected and inevitable, we see ourselves as all walking the same path. With this empathy, we have the power to work together, to continue to improve our communities to be more welcoming, easier to navigate, and more inclusive of those who don't fit the narrow definition of normal. Perhaps this empathy is the most advanced parenting skill of all.

Acknowledgments

This book has been a passion project. For years I have seen some parents struggle to access resources for their children simply because they had less knowledge and experience navigating health and educational systems. When I had cancer as a child, I directly benefited from my parents' advocacy. Certainly, we had it easier than many because of the privilege of having financial and educational resources at our disposal, but my mother had also learned a lot the hard way when her brother faced childhood cancer. Her sophistication in facing my challenge and earned knowledge of how to navigate the health-care system has been an inspiration. Thanks to my mom and dad for relentlessly advocating for me.

I can't be everyone's doctor nor can I even give advice to all the people who follow me on social media. But as I observed this struggle as a physician, I said to myself, "What if I could try to narrow this gap and help parents learn the skills they need to support their children in a challenge?" I am so thankful to the many friends and colleagues who fueled this passion and encouraged me to give it a try.

Many role models in medicine were particularly helpful. My oncologist Dr. Joanne Kurtzberg inspired me with her kindness and knowledge. My residency mentors Dr. Andrew Racine, Dr. Miriam Schechter, and Dr. Peter Belamarich helped me see how my varied interests didn't quite fit into any one path within academia, planting the seeds that would later blossom into this book. My complex care colleagues Dr. Alex Okun, Dr. Ruth Stein, Dr. Sarah Norris, Dr. Kristina Malik, and Dr. Kathryn Scharbach taught me so much about how to approach and provide best care for families with more serious illness. Dr. Hina Talib has been a friend and cheerleader—I'm thankful for her support and not sure I would have gotten this book done without her.

Additionally, I would like to thank the Women Physician Writers and the SoMeDocs community for inspiration and guidance. While social media is not without its problems, I have found it to be such an incredible resource to connect with others with shared interests. Thank you to my more experienced writer friends Emily Oster, Lauren Smith Brody, Pooja Lakshmin, Melinda Moyer, Tina Payne Bryson, and Virginia Sole-Smith for being open to connecting with me and sharing your wisdom. Your support and guidance have been essential as I brought this book to life.

Thank you to Craig Canapari, a fellow physician author for believing in my idea and introducing me to my agent. I am so appreciative to have Celeste Fine in my corner—she immediately saw the importance of this topic and has been an essential thought partner in bringing it to life. Thank you to Nana K. Twumasi and the Balance imprint at Grand Central Publishing of Hachette for your tireless efforts and patience as we shaped a rough manuscript into what you see today. Thanks also to Emi Ikkanda for additional editorial support and pushing me to address the gender equity issues central to caregiving parents.

As I wrote and edited this book, I relied on many experts to share their stories—parents educators and medical providers, including Dr. Helen Egger, Caitlin Murray, Caroline Cook, Courtney Aseltine, Dr. David Stukus, Debbie Cohen, Deborah Vilas, Emily Holl, Erin F., Erin (@FoodScienceBabe), Hannah Heck, Priscilla and Abigail Jean Baptiste, Jon Rosenshine, Laura Vanderkam, Meghan Marsac, Theresa J., and Virginia Sole-Smith. Many of these individuals consented to publicly sharing their stories and our discussions have been released as a podcast. Each of their stories and their perspectives enriched this work in meaningful ways.

Truly, I have learned something from each family I have worked with as a pediatrician. Some families have allowed me to peek behind the curtain and see more than what most pediatricians typically see. It is an honor and a privilege to have this sort of trust with families during very fragile and tumultuous times in their lives. While all the stories shared in this book are heavily anonymized—names, genders, ages, and diagnoses shifted around—I hope I have done justice to the realities of family life. Thanks also to the content creators in the children's disability community who have so eloquently shared their perspective to further enhance my understanding and respect for their experiences.

When I decided to write this book, I was between jobs due to the pandemic. I had no idea what I was getting myself into and that I might be launching a new practice while finalizing the book. Without the encouragement and support of some of my closest friends, I'm not sure I would have gotten it done. Thank you to my friends, especially Diana Gershuny (my unofficial publicist!), Alli Chiaramonte, and Kate Piekarski for always encouraging me to just keep swimming. Thanks also to Laura, Vicky, Kate, Stacey, Gavitt, and Lyndsey for our decades of friendship.

Most importantly, I'd like to thank my husband, Bill, who believed in me and my ability to be more than *just* a pediatrician years before I even voiced the idea to anyone else. Without his unconditional support and encouragement, this book would not be here. Additionally, while I don't talk about our co-parenting much in the books I've written, he is the best partner I could ask for in raising our incredible children—and this book would not have been written without his assistance with childcare and meal preparation. He's the best; nobody beats him. Thanks to my children for teaching me more about caring for children than I ever learned in training.

Resources

There are hundreds of resources that might be helpful for your family. Without knowing where you are or your unique situation, it's impossible for me to guess which might be the most relevant. Here I've included some of the most impactful organizations nationally.

- **Family Voices:** The mission of Family Voices is to promote health equity and improve services for children with special health-care needs and disabilities. They have supported many programs and projects over the years, some of which are ongoing such as the Youth as Self Advocates (YASA) program.
- **Courageous Parents Network (CPN):** Courageous Parents Network aims to support and empower families caring for children with serious illnesses. They have programs and services as well as a free library of videos, podcasts, and guides.
- **Variety, the Children's Charity:** Variety is an international organization that serves children with disabilities and serious illnesses. In the US, they have three programs through which they provide medical, mobility, and communication equipment and services to individual children as well as organizations. Programs vary internationally, but with the main mission of serving children in need being the same.
- **Lucile Packard Foundation for Children's Health:** The David and Lucile Packard Foundation has a program to address the national needs of the 20 percent of children in the US who have a special health-care need. They work to improve the lives of children,

families, and communities by improving the quality and accessibility of health care.

- **Make-A-Wish:** Make-A-Wish grants wishes to children diagnosed with critical illnesses. By doing so, they hope to raise the spirits of children and their families to give them hope and the strength to continue fighting their illnesses.

- **SeriousFun Children's Network:** SeriousFun Children's Network provides a safe and inclusive camp experience for kids with serious illnesses. Their camp programs were designed to foster independence, promote self-confidence, build community, and help empower children so they can see beyond the limits of their medical condition. There are thirty camps and programs located around the world.

- **Ronald McDonald House Charities:** The Ronald McDonald House Charities have three core programs. The most well-known of their programs provides families with a home-like place to stay close to the hospital where their child is receiving care. They also have the Ronald McDonald Family Room, which provides a quiet space in the hospital where families can recharge, eat, sleep, and shower. They also have a mobile health program that provides dental and medical services to underserved communities.

- **Sibling Support Project:** The Sibling Support Project is a program for the brothers and sisters of children with special needs. They provide support for siblings through online communities and through Sibshops, which are events for siblings to connect with each other while also having fun. Sibshops are all across the US and Canada and many other countries as well.

- **Easterseals:** Easterseals works toward equity and inclusion for people with disabilities of all ages. They provide services and support through their many programs, which include autism services, transportation services, in-home care, camping and recreation programs, and much more.

- **Eye to Eye:** Eye to Eye provides programs and services for kids with learning disabilities and differences (such as those with ADHD), as well as courses for educators to help them better understand the needs of their students with learning differences. Eye to Eye is unique in that it is also run by people with learning differences, and all mentors in their programs also have learning differences. There are twenty different locations within the US.
- **Creative Healing for Youth in Pain (CHYP):** CHYP is an online non-profit for youth with chronic pain and their parents, providing information, self-help tools, social support, and creative arts experiences.

Mental Health

If you're looking to learn more about some of the mental health conditions I mentioned, these resources are a good place to start.

- **National Child Traumatic Stress Network (NCTSN):** The NCTSN aims to increase access to services for children and their families who have experienced or witnessed traumatic events. It was created in 2000 by Congress as part of the Children's Health Act. Their website has guides for families and caregivers to help children process traumatic events. Additionally, NCTSN Learning Center offers free online education and courses.
- **National Alliance on Mental Illness (NAMI):** NAMI provides education and support for people and families affected by mental illness. The resources they provide include classes, a toll-free helpline, and support groups.
- **Child Mind Institute:** The mission of Child Mind Institute is to improve the lives of the millions of children in the US struggling with mental health and learning challenges. They have science/research programs to help discover new and innovative treatments and several

educational programs for both children and their families. Their website has a Family Resource Center for parents and caretakers that includes a symptom checker, a resource finder, parenting guides, and more. They also provide care both in person (New York City and Bay Area) and through telehealth (New York, New Jersey, California).

- **MentalHealth.gov:** MentalHealth.gov has a lot of information on their site about different mental health conditions. There are guides for young people, parents, educators, and others on how to deal with mental health issues as well as info on how to access various help lines such as the Suicide & Crisis Lifeline.

If you need help finding therapy, or are having trouble finding therapy you can afford, try the resources listed below:

- Federally Qualified Health Centers
- Substance Abuse and Mental Health Services Administration
- American Psychoanalytic Association
- Mental Health America
- Psychology Today

If you are looking for telemedicine alternatives to improve your ability to access care, try these:

- GoodTherapy
- Brightline
- Little Otter
- Talkspace

If you need help affording prescription medicine, there are many programs available:

- Coupon services like GoodRx, SingleCare, America's Pharmacy, ScriptSave WellRx, and Optum Perks.

- Retailers including Walmart, Costco, Walgreens, and Amazon Prime all offer programs.
- NeedyMeds, RxHope, RxAssist, and Patient Assistance help connect families with pharmaceutical companies for patient-assistance programs.

Further Reading

Communication, Time Management, and Decision-Making

Faber, A. & Mazlish, E. 2012. *How to Talk So Kids Will Listen & Listen So Kids Will Talk*. New York: Scribner.

Oster, E. 2021. *The Family Firm: A Data-Driven Guide to Better Decision Making in the Early School Years*. New York: Penguin Press.

Rodsky, E. 2019. *Fair Play: A Game-Changing Solution for When You Have Too Much to Do (and More Life to Live)*. New York: G.P. Putnam's Sons.

On Parenting Children with Differences

Biel, L. & Peske, N. 2018. *Raising a Sensory Smart Child: The Definitive Handbook for Helping Your Child with Sensory Processing Issues*. New York: Penguin Books.

Franklin, D. & Cozolino, L. 2018. *Helping Your Child with Language-Based Learning Disabilities: Strategies to Succeed in School and Life with Dyslexia, Dysgraphia, Dyscalculia, ADHD, and Processing Disorders*. Oakland: New Harbinger Publications.

Klass, P. & Costello, E. 2021. *Quirky Kids: Understanding and Supporting Your Child with Developmental Differences*. Itasca: American Academy of Pediatrics.

Kurcinka, M. S. 2015. *Raising Your Spirited Child: A Guide for Parents Whose Child Is More Intense, Sensitive, Perceptive, Persistent, and Energetic*. 3rd ed. New York: William Morrow Paperbacks.

Lebowitz, E. 2020. *Breaking Free of Child Anxiety and OCD: A Scientifically Proven Program for Parents*. Oxford: Oxford University Press.

Marsac, M. & Hogan, M. 2021. *Afraid of the Doctor: Every Parent's Guide to Preventing and Managing Medical Trauma*. Lanham: Rowman & Littlefield Publishers.

Solomon, A. 2013. *Far from the Tree: Parents, Children and the Search for Identity*. New York: Scribner.

Selected Memoirs from Parents of Children with Special Health-Care Needs

Brown, I. 2011. *The Boy in the Moon: A Father's Journey to Understand His Extraordinary Son*. New York: St. Martin's Press.

Lanier, H. 2020. *Raising a Rare Girl: A Memoir*. New York: Penguin Books.

Lee, K. J. 2021. *Catastrophic Rupture: A Memoir of Healing*. Waukesha: Ten16 Press.

Sleep

Canapari, C. 2019. "It's never too late to sleep train," in *The Low-Stress Way to High-Quality Sleep for Babies, Kids, and Parents*. New York: Rodale Books.

Huffington, A. 2016. *The Sleep Revolution: Transforming Your Life, One Night at a Time*. New York: Harmony.

Weissbluth, M. 2015. *Healthy Sleep Habits, Happy Child: A Step-by-Step Program for a Good Night's Sleep*. 4th ed. New York: Ballantine Books.

Siblings

Faber, A. & Mazlish, E. 2012. *Siblings Without Rivalry: How to Help Your Children Live Together So You Can Live Too*. New York: Norton.

Strohm, K. 2005. *Being the Other One: Growing Up with a Brother or Sister Who Has Special Needs*. Boulder: Shambhala.

Notes

Chapter 1: *Understanding Your Reaction to a Problem*

1. Lynch-Jordan, A. M. et al. 2013. "The interplay of parent and adolescent catastrophizing and its impact on adolescent pain, functioning, and pain behavior." *Clinical Journal of Pain* 29(8): 681–688.
2. Because the medical community has such a history of marginalizing individuals with chronic pain, I want to clarify that this doesn't imply that parents cause their child's pain or the pain is not real. Chronic pain is absolutely real, and it's essential to have a comprehensive treatment plan, including all potentially helpful treatments from pain medication and adjunctive measures such as acupuncture to behavioral health interventions to treat anxiety, depression, and perhaps reduce tendency toward catastrophizing. For more information, a great resource to learn more is the nonprofit Creative Healing for Youth in Pain (mychyp.org).
3. Pinquart, M. 2018. "Parenting stress in caregivers of children with chronic physical condition—a meta-analysis." *Stress Health* 34(2):197–207.
4. Kim, H. et al. 2021. "Internalizing psychopathology and all-cause mortality: A comparison of transdiagnostic vs. diagnosis-based risk prediction." *World Psychiatry* 20(2): 276–282.
5. May, R. 1963. "Freedom and responsibility reexamined" in *Behavioral Science and Guidance: Proposals and Perspectives*, edited by Esther Lloyd-Jones and Esther M. Westervelt, pp. 101–102. New York: Bureau of Publications, Teachers College, Columbia University.

Chapter 2: *What Matters Most?*

1. While President Dwight Eisenhower invented the matrix, it was popularized by Stephen Covey in his book *The 7 Habits of Highly Effective People*.
2. Astill, R. G. et al. 2012. "Sleep, cognition, and behavioral problems in school-age children: A century of research meta-analyzed." *Psychological Bulletin* 138(6): 1109–1138.
3. Kiris, M. et al. 2010. "Changes in serum IGF-1 and IGFBP-3 levels and growth in children following adenoidectomy, tonsillectomy or adenotonsillectomy." *International Journal of Pediatric Otorhinolaryngology* 74(5): 528–531.
4. Hartley, J. et al. 2021. "The physical health of caregivers of children with life-limiting conditions: A systematic review." *Pediatrics* 148(2): 1.

5. Li, L. et al. 2016. "Insomnia and the risk of depression: A meta-analysis of prospective cohort studies." *BMC Psychiatry* 16(1): 375.

6. Grandner, M.A. et al. 2016. "Sleep: Important considerations for the prevention of cardiovascular disease." *Current Opinion in Cardiology* 31(5): 551–565.

7. Grandner, M. A. et al. 2016. "Sleep duration and diabetes risk: Population trends and potential mechanisms." *Current Diabetes Reports* 16(11): 106.

8. Colten, H. R. & Altevogt, B. M., eds. 2006. *Sleep Disorders and Sleep Deprivation: An Unmet Public Health Problem*. Board on Health Sciences Policy; National Academies Press.

9. Cohen, S. et al. 2009. "Sleep habits and susceptibility to the common cold." *Archives of Internal Medicine* 169(1): 62–67.

10. Hudson, A. N., Van Dongen, H. P. A., & Honn, K. A. 2020. "Sleep deprivation, vigilant attention, and brain function: A review." *Neuropsychopharmacology* 45(1): 21–30.

11. McEwen, B. S. & Karatsoreos, I. N. 2015. "Sleep deprivation and circadian disruption: Stress, allostasis, and allostatic load." *Sleep Medicine Clinics* 10(1): 1–10.

12. In 2012, the *Lancet* developed an international working group and published an entire issue devoted to the importance of physical activity for health and well-being. All the pieces are relevant, especially the following: Kohl, H. W. III et al. 2012. "The pandemic of physical inactivity: Global action for public health." *Lancet*, Physical Activity Series Working Group 380(9838): 294–305.

13. Ho, C. L., Wu, W. F., & Liou, Y. M. 2019. "Dose-response relationship of outdoor exposure and myopia indicators: A systematic review and meta-analysis of various research methods." *International Journal of Environmental Research and Public Health* 16(14): 2595.

14. Fyfe-Johnson, A. L. et al. 2021. "Nature and children's health: A systematic review." *Pediatrics* 148 (4): 1.

15. Murphy, J. M. et al. 1998. "The relationship of school breakfast to psychosocial and academic functioning: Cross-sectional and longitudinal observations in an inner-city school sample." *Archives of Pediatrics and Adolescent Medicine* 152(9): 899–907.

16. Greening, L. et al. 2007. "Child routines and youth adherence to treatment for type 1 diabetes." *Journal of Pediatric Psychology* 32(4): 437–447.

17. Grossoehme, D. H., Filigno, S. S., & Bishop, M. 2014. "Parent routines for managing cystic fibrosis in children." *Journal of Clinical Psychology in Medical Settings* 21(2): 125–135.

18. Bates, C. R. et al. 2021. "Family rules, routines, and caregiver distress during the first year of pediatric cancer treatment." *Psychooncology* 30(9): 1590–1599.

19. Bethell, C. et al. 2019. "Positive childhood experiences and adult mental and relational health in a statewide sample: Associations across adverse childhood experiences levels." *JAMA Pediatrics* 173(11): e193007.

20. Garwick, A. W. et al. 1998. "Family recommendations for improving services for children with chronic conditions." *Archives of Pediatric and Adolescent Medicine* 152(5): 440–448.

Chapter 3: *Medical and Educational Literacy*

1. The CDC maintains an excellent website summarizing the impact of social determinants of health, as they are priorities to address for public health initiatives. This report published in March 2022 is an excellent primer:
"Health Equity and Health Disparities Environmental Scan." 2022. Rockville, MD: US Department of Health and Human Services, Office of the Assistant Secretary for Health, Office of Disease Prevention and Health Promotion.
2. Bocian, A. B. et al. 1999. "Size and age-sex distribution of pediatric practice: A study from Pediatric Research in Office Settings." *Archives of Pediatric and Adolescent Medicine* 153(1): 9–14.
3. Osterberg, L. & Blaschke, T. 2005. "Adherence to medication." *New England Journal of Medicine* 353(5): 487–497.
4. Medication nonadherence causes at least 125,000 preventable deaths a year and nearly $100 billion in preventable medical costs. Kleinsinger, F. 2018. "The unmet challenge of medication nonadherence." *Permanente Journal* 22:18–33.
5. Though many articles have examined this in children and more specific subgroups, impressive evidence about this can be reviewed here:
Birkmeyer, J. D. et al. 2002. "Hospital volume and surgical mortality in the United States." *New England Journal of Medicine* 346(15): 1128–1137.
Jenkins, K. J. et al. 1995. "In-hospital mortality for surgical repair of congenital heart defects: Preliminary observations of variation by hospital caseload." *Pediatrics* 95(3): 323-330.
6. Whitney, D. G. & Peterson, M. D. 2019. "US national and state-level prevalence of mental health disorders and disparities of mental health care use in children." *JAMA Pediatrics* 173(4): 389–391.
7. Howard, K. I. et al. 1986. "The dose–effect relationship in psychotherapy." *American Psychologist* 41(2): 159–164.
8. Brooks, S. J. & Stein, D. J. 2015. "A systematic review of the neural bases of psychotherapy for anxiety and related disorders." *Dialogues in Clinical Neuroscience* 17(3): 261–279.
9. This data is compiled from the National Center for Education Statistics and updated at https://nces.ed.gov/programs/coe/indicator/cgg.

Chapter 4: *Understanding the Bigger Picture*

1. If this is your challenge, I'd highly recommend exploring Eli Lebowitz's great book *Breaking Free of Child Anxiety and OCD*.
2. To learn more about the process of care mapping, I suggest you investigate the resources from Boston Children's Hospital and Children's Wisconsin. If you prefer academic resources, you can read more here: Adams, S. et al. 2017. "Care maps for children with medical complexity." *Developmental Medicine and Child Neurology* 59(12): 1299–1306.

Chapter 5: *Educating Yourself*

1. For more details on how to evaluate health information online, check out this tutorial developed by the National Library of Medicine: https://medlineplus.gov /webeval/EvaluatingInternetHealthInformationTutorial.pdf.

Chapter 6: *Tools, Skills, and Tips to Build You Up*

1. A recent article, "How same-sex couples divide chores, and what it reveals about modern parenting" by Claire Cain Miller in the *New York Times* describes this in more detail.
2. Daminger, A. 2019. "The cognitive dimension of household labor." *American Sociological Review* 84(4): 609–633.
3. This study is relatively small and from 2007, but it's surprisingly difficult to find more recent national data about who takes children to the doctor.
   Cox, E. D. et al. 2007. "Effect of gender and visit length on participation in pediatric visits." *Patient Education and Counseling* 65(3): 320–328.
4. Urkin, J. et al. 2008. "Who accompanies a child to the office of the physician?" *International Journal of Adolescent Medicine and Health* 20(4): 513–518.
5. Daly, M. & Groes, F. 2017. "Who takes the child to the doctor? Mom, pretty much all of the time." *Applied Economics Letters* 24: 1267–1276.
6. To read more about the need for research about paternal postpartum depression, see this article:
   Walsh, T. B., Davis, R. N., & Garfield, C. 2020. "A call to action: Screening fathers for perinatal depression." *Pediatrics* 145(1): e20191193.
7. Yogman, M. et al. 2016. "Fathers' roles in the care and development of their children: The role of pediatricians." *Pediatrics* 138 (1): e20161128.
8. If you want to take the next steps to make change happen within your family, Eve Rodsky's *Fair Play* book is a great guide for starting a conversation with your partner. To understand the bigger picture of work-family justice, Brigid Schulte's Better Life Lab has a podcast and newsletter where you can learn more about opportunities to advocate for paid leave, improvements to childcare policies, and changes in the workplace that can support equity within families.
9. To read more about the social science research behind goal-setting and task motivation, I highly recommend this article:
   Locke, E. A. & Latham, G. P. 2002. "Building a practically useful theory of goal setting and task motivation. A 35-year odyssey." *American Psychologist* 57(9): 705–717.
10. In case you are curious, febrile seizures are brief, generalized, self-resolving seizures that accompany high fevers in children six months to five years of age. While they can be very scary to experience, they often do not indicate an underlying diagnosis like epilepsy or pose a long-term risk to the child.
11. When discarding medications, consider the safest way to do so and ask your pharmacist. Some communities have take-back programs. The FDA recommends flushing controlled substances down the toilet. For other medications, it's recommended to mix them with something unappetizing like dirt or coffee grounds, place them in a sealed container, and then discard in the trash.

Chapter 7: *Taking Inventory of the Rest of Your Family*

1. Sharpe, D. & Rossiter, L. 2002. "Siblings of children with a chronic illness: A meta-analysis." *Journal of Pediatric Psychology* 27(8): 699–710.

Chapter 8: *Respecting Your Child's Space and Development*

1. Got Transition is a federally funded national resource center aiming to improve health-care transitions.
2. Kessels, R. P. 2003. "Patients' memory for medical information." *Journal of the Royal Society of Medicine* 96(5): 219–222.
3. To further explore family communication plans and meetings, I'd recommend the book *The Secrets of Happy Families* by Bruce Feiler.
4. *How to Talk So Kids Will Listen & Listen So Kids Will Talk* by Adele Faber and Elaine Mazlish has many great ideas for improving communication with kids.

Chapter 9: *Confronting Hard Feelings and Burnout*

1. This essay has been helpful for many parents facing a challenge, normalizing the experience of mixed feelings regarding your child's challenge. But it's important to acknowledge this perspective is not the *only* special-needs parent experience. Joy can be extraordinarily difficult to find if your child is demonstrating violent behavior or a painful life-limiting condition. As unique as a child's challenge may be, parents are entitled to experience their child's diagnosis in their own way too.
2. Coller, R. J. et al. 2016. "Medical complexity among children with special health care needs: A two-dimensional view." *Health Services Research* 51(4): 1644–1669.
3. Guidi, J. et al. 2021. "Allostatic load and its impact on health: A systematic review." *Psychotherapy and Psychosomatics* 90(1): 11–27.
4. Zimmer, B. 2017. "The Chinese origins of 'paper tiger.'" Retrieved from: https://www.wsj.com/articles/the-chinese-origins-of-paper-tiger-1487873046.
5. Wang, H., Cui, H., Wang, M., & Yang, C. 2021. "What you believe can affect how you feel: Anger among caregivers of elderly people with dementia." *Frontiers of Psychiatry* 12: 633730.
6. Sullivan, P. M. & Knutson, J. F. 2000. "Maltreatment and disabilities: a population-based epidemiological study." *Child Abuse and Neglect* 24(10): 1257–1273.
7. Hassmén, P., Koivula, N., & Uutela, A. 2000. "Physical exercise and psychological well-being: a population study in Finland." *Preventative Medicine* 30(1): 17–25.
8. Kammerer, A. 2019. "Scientific underpinnings and impacts of shame." *Scientific American.*
9. Lindström, C., Aman, J., & Norberg, A. L. 2010. "Increased prevalence of burnout symptoms in parents of chronically ill children." *Acta Paediatrica* 99(3): 427–432.
10. In the Women's Health Initiative, they tracked 97,253 women over time and found that cynicism was related to higher risk of death.
11. In the *New York Times*, Dr. Lakshmin wrote an article entitled "How society has turned its back on mothers," which can be viewed at https://www.nytimes

.com/2021/02/04/parenting/working-mom-burnout-coronavirus.html. To be fair, while mothers statistically carry more caregiving and parenting duties, fathers can also feel betrayed by the level of stress they carry in this work.

12. David, D., Cristea, I., & Hofmann, S. G. 2018. "Why cognitive behavioral therapy is the current gold standard of psychotherapy." *Front Psychiatry* 9: 4.

13. Eccleston, C. et al. 2015. "Psychological interventions for parents of children and adolescents with chronic illness." *Cochrane Database of Systematic Reviews* 4(4): CD009660. Update in: *Cochrane Database of Systematic Rev*iews 2019, 2021(6): CD009660.

14. Cousineau, T. M., Hobbs, L. M., & Arthur, K. C. 2019. "The role of compassion and mindfulness in building parental resilience when caring for children with chronic conditions: A conceptual model." *Frontiers in Psychology* 10: 1602.

15. Nguyen, J. & Brymer, E. 2018. "Nature-based guided imagery as an intervention for state anxiety." *Frontiers in Psychology* 9: 1858.

16. Slimani, M. et al. 2016. "Effects of mental imagery on muscular strength in healthy and patient participants: A systematic review." *Journal of Sports Science & Medicine* 15(3): 434–450.

17. Zaccaro, A. et al. 2018. "How breath-control can change your life: A systematic review on psycho-physiological correlates of slow breathing." *Frontiers in Human Neuroscience* 12: 353.

Chapter 10: *Understanding Your Child's Resistance*

1. Based on the diagnostic criteria for generalized anxiety disorder listed in the American Psychiatric Association, *Diagnostic and Statistical Manual of Mental Disorders*, Fifth Edition (DSM-5), American Psychiatric Association, Arlington, VA 2013.

2. Bennett, S. et al. 2015. "Psychological interventions for mental health disorders in children with chronic physical illness: a systematic review." *Archives of Disease in Childhood* 100(4): 308–316.

3. Extrapolated from the diagnostic criteria for depression listed in the American Psychiatric Association, *Diagnostic and Statistical Manual of Mental Disorders*, Fifth Edition (DSM-5), American Psychiatric Association, Arlington, VA 2013.

Chapter 11: *Unpacking Trauma and Protecting Joy*

1. To learn more about the evidence-based approaches to treating trauma, explore resources within the National Child Traumatic Stress Network. Many of the summaries of treatment options that follow are reviewed in more detail on their website.

2. Louie, D., Brook, K., & Frates, E. 2016. "The laughter prescription: A tool for lifestyle medicine." *American Journal of Lifestyle Medicine* 10(4): 262–267.

3. Brown, B. 2013, updated 2017. "The fast track to genuine joy." *HuffPost.* Retrieved from https://www.huffpost.com/entry/finding-happiness-brene-brown_n _4312653.

Chapter 12: *Making a Comprehensive Plan*

1. The AAP has a comprehensive policy statement about school safety that reviews a number of conditions, including food allergy, here:
   Gereige, R. S., Gross, T., & Jastaniah, E. 2022. "Individual medical emergencies occurring at school." *Pediatrics* 150(1): 1.
2. You can read more about the Emergency Information Form at this website: https://www.acep.org/by-medical-focus/pediatrics/medical-forms/emergency-information-form-for-children-with-special-health-care-needs/.

Chapter 13: *Maintaining Motivation*

1. For a deeper discussion about cultivating motivation, I recommend reading *The Self-Driven Child* by William Stixrud and Ned Johnson.

Index

About the Author

Dr. Kelly Fradin is a pediatrician and passionate advocate for children and parents. Originally from Charlotte, North Carolina, she was inspired to become a doctor by her experience surviving childhood cancer. As a pediatrician, she has spent her career working with families in academic complex care, public health–oriented school programs, and private practice. Her first book *Parenting in a Pandemic: How to Help Your Family through COVID-19* helped to inform and empower parents during difficult times. She shares advice on social media @AdviceIGive MyFriends. Kelly lives with her husband, Bill, and her two children in New York City.